Creating What's Next

✳✳✳✳✳✳

Gracefully

Other books by Valerie Ramsey:

Gracefully: Looking and Being Your Best at Any Age

*"**Gracefully** is simply wonderful. Valerie Ramsey is living proof that being older than fifty can be exciting, healthy, and sexy."*

- CHRISTIANE NORTHRUP, M.D.—author of *Mother-Daughter Wisdom, The Wisdom of Menopause, and Women's Bodies, Women's Wisdom*

"Valerie Ramsey is the new face, style, and attitude of aging. In *Gracefully*, she inspires us to bring out the best in ourselves—physically, mentally, and spiritually—in order to make the fifty-plus years the best years of our lives. A terrific, uplifting, and informative book."

- KEN DYCHTWALD, Ph.D., president and CEO of Age Wave and author of *Bodymind, Healthy Aging, The Age Wave,* and *The Power Years.*

"I like the snappy way this gal thinks. She sends out a powerful message!"

- RUE McCLANAHAN, Emmy Award-winning actress and author of *My First Five Husbands... and the Ones Who Got Away*

Creating What's Next

✽ ✽ ✽ ✽ ✽ ✽

Gracefully

Valerie Ramsey

With Heather Hummel

PathBinder Publishing

Library of Congress Cataloging-in-Publication Data

Ramsey, Valerie. Creating What's Next: Gracefully
by Valerie Ramsey with Heather Hummel p.cm.

ISBN 9 780988 225091
   1. Life skills—Handbooks, manuals, etc.
   2. Aging—Handbooks, manuals, etc. I. Hummel,
Heather.
   II. Title.

ISBN 9 780988 225091
Interior design by Heather Hummel
Photographs on part openers and Chapters 1, 2, 3, 5, 8, 10, 17 copyright
© by Deidre Fuller; on Chapter 6, 11, 12 copyright ©
by Tom O'Neal TGO Photography; on Chapter 7
copyright © by Bill Janes; on Chapter 9 copyright ©
by Roberto Ligresti; on Chapters 18 and Foreword
with Ali MacGraw from the personal collection of
the author; on Chapter 13 copyright © by Style
Magazine; on Part Two © Christine Rose; on Chapter
16, 17 © Scott Campbell; on Part One © Deidre Fuller

The information contained in this book is intended
to provide helpful and informative material on the
subject addressed. It is not intended to serve as a
replacement for professional medical advice. Any use
of the information in this book is at the reader's
discretion. The author and publisher specifically
disclaim any and all liability arising directly or
indirectly from the use or application of any
information contained in this book. A healthcare
professional should be consulted regarding your
specific situation.

Dedication

To Mima and Poppy

Table of Contents

$\mathcal{F}$oreword
by Ali MacGraw

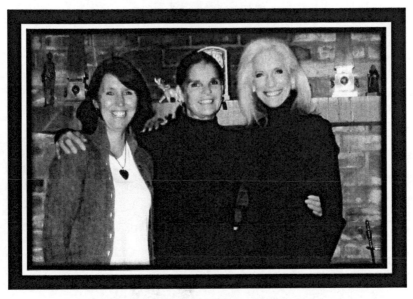

Heather Hummel, Ali MacGraw, Valerie Ramsey
Carmel, CA 2010

I love it when our lives circle back around and reconnect us with people who were important to us in the past. This is what happened for me when, after many years and different geographies and lives, I met again with one of my friends who was really important to me in our high school days. I had admired and loved Valerie Ramsey throughout our school years, and we had lost touch somehow; and now she has reappeared as a beautiful and wise Mother, Wife, Grandmother, Model and Inspirational Speaker... a real inspiration for women of our age, and the same lovely human being that she had always been. "Creating What's Next - Gracefully" is her second book, and it is written with the same candor and clarity and Heart that defined her when we were both teenagers... only now, there is real wisdom to share. Above all, this book radiates Optimism and Joy, and serves as one of those blueprints for those of us women who keep reinventing ourselves and seizing, with enthusiasm and Grace, "What's Next."

Introduction

An incredible time awaits us when we can go through life, eager to discover new ways to make the journey ever more exciting, ever more adventuresome, and ever more fulfilling. When I first wrote *Gracefully—Looking and Being Your Best at Any Age*—I had just come through a major crossroads in my life. Not only was I a middle-aged woman with an empty nest, but I had also faced two life threatening health challenges—one with heart disease, the other with cancer. This is the story of how I persevered and emerged on the other side of that dark tunnel a victor - thrilled to have discovered that if you live your life with joy and vitality, have a positive attitude and an open mind, life can just get better and better. Being your best self in body, mind and spirit was the focus of *Gracefully*.

This book begins with the premise that in order to create What's Next, it is imperative that you feel and look your best—so that you are already starting off on a solid foundation. Therefore, you will see that Part One offers some of the same core principles (with updates) on living a fit, young and vital life as my first book had.

Part Two is all about recognizing and creating your own What's Next. It answers questions such as *How do I know what I want to do next*? What do I do if a great opportunity drops in my lap, but I'm afraid to go after it? What if I don't have the courage? The confidence? The know-how? How do I know which opportunity is right for me? What do I do if I'm forced to make a transition, but I have no idea what it should be? How do I move past the fear and breathe in success? How do I go after something I want? How do I stay strong mentally, physically, spiritually? I answer all of these questions—and more—because my answers evolved when I faced them myself. I was determined that the second half of my life was going to be just as magnificent as the first half had been, and I was going to do whatever it took to make it that way, both personally and professionally.

Today I am still flying high on this wondrous adventure called Life, knowing that there are a host of new experiences and new opportunities waiting just around the corner. I smile to myself, happy and thrilled, that the secrets to uncovering them lie within my being, and that now I can share them with you. I can't wait to tell you how I did it and how you can too!

Acknowledgements

Acknowledgements are nice—they serve an important purpose for anyone who has ever authored a book, but acknowledging those who have played such an important part in helping me to write this book, isn't nearly enough. There is so much more I want to say. I want to begin by thanking the major contributors to *Creating What's Next–Gracefully*. When I first set out on this project, a large part of it was designed to give the reader updated information on the subjects of sleep, nutrition, healthy aging and sexuality from the top authorities who had contributed so heavily to my first book.

When I started thinking about writing this book, I began by calling each one of you to ask if you would mind giving me updated contributions. You were all so gracious in responding to my request for assistance the second time around; therefore, let me begin by saying a very big Thank You and expressing my heartfelt appreciation to Dr. Michael Breus, PhD, for your invaluable help on Advice From the Sleep Doctor, to Derek Johnson for the help you always so graciously give me on Nutrition, to Arlene Noodleman, MD, and Bruce Berman, MD, for your contributions to the chapter on Healthy Aging; to Ashley Solomon, Psy.D, who so generously shared her wisdom on what mindful exercise is all about, and to my dear friend, Lou Paget, who so beautifully demystifies all of our questions on Sexuality. You all have been so generous with your time and expertise. Saying Thank You doesn't begin to tell you how appreciative I am, but to each of you—a warm and very heartfelt Thank You.

To my good friend, literary agent and editor, Olga Vezeris—what would I ever do without you? You are the Best in every way, and I couldn't have done this without your help. Your wisdom and guidance have been key to this project. Thank you.

One of the greatest gifts we have in this life is the real friends we make along the way—people who come into our lives and make such an imprint on our hearts and souls that they are a part of us forever. Ali MacGraw is one of those friends in my life. Ali, you are one of the kindest, most generous, loving and warm-hearted women it has ever been my joy and privilege to know. Having you in my life for all these years has been like a bright and shining star out there in the Heavens, not always visible, but always constant. You were so dear to write the foreword for this book in spite of your incredibly busy schedule, and I love and appreciate you for your thoughtfulness more than I can say. It is an honor to have you be a part of this project. Thank you.

To my talented and beautiful daughter, Heather... If it weren't for you, neither *Gracefully* nor this book would ever have been written. You have helped your mom every step of the way, from concept to cover design, to writing and publishing, and I am so very grateful for your love, your support, your professionalism, your amazing talent, and your invaluable help. Thank you.

To my incredible family, starting with my loving, supportive husband of fifty-three years, Wally. You have been my number one cheerleader all along the way. You have put up with countless hours of seeing the back of my head as I sat glued to my computer—laughing and joking to keep me going—but never complaining. Thank you for your love, your divine patience, and your cheerful support in everything I do. You are always behind me, and I love you for it. Thank you!

And to the rest of our wonderful family—Jim, Darcy, Annie, Gus and Katy—you bring your Dad and me such joy and happiness every single day, and having your loving support as I wrote this book meant the world to me. Thank you, each and every one.

I am not finished there, however, because there are eight grandchildren who light up my life and who make me smile every time I think of them. Through the most challenging times as I wrote this book (and as we all know, writing can be a difficult and solitary process), just thinking of your happy faces made me smile and kept me going. Having you in our lives means everything. I send warm hugs to Kristin, PJ, our two Jacks, Matthew, Lauren, Alex and Jennifer. I love you all.

Friends and loved ones are what life is all about, and so I want to conclude by first of all, thanking my new and fabulously talented friend, Minx Boren, for all of the ways you enrich my life, right down to your beautiful poetry. Having two of your writings included in this book is such an honor.

And finally, to all of the friends who have been such an important part of my life everywhere Wally and I have lived —knowing you are out there means the world to me. To all of the wonderful new friends I've made since moving to south Florida—I have been overwhelmed by your warmth and kindness. It's no wonder that I fall more in love with this area every single day.

My heartfelt appreciation to you all.

Love,

Valerie

PART ONE

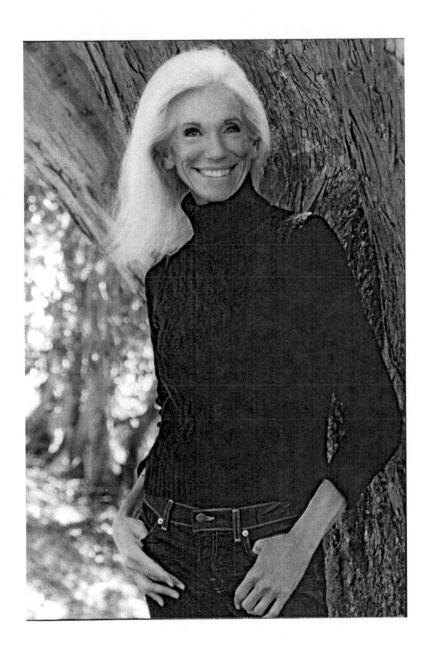

CHAPTER 1: Hello, Beautiful!

Beauty Is The Vitality That Shines From Within

— Valerie Ramsey

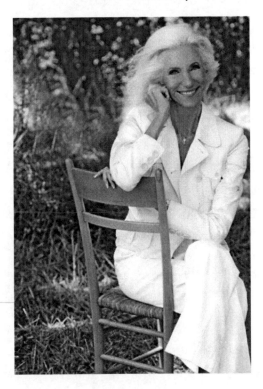

When you are reading through Part One of this book, it may feel like familiar territory. That is because there are certain core elements from *Gracefully—Looking and Being Your Best at Any Age* that are just as important today as they were five years ago. However, you will also see that there is a lot of new material. For example, the chapter on nutrition comes with brand new information from my nutritionist in Los Angeles, Derek Johnson, of New Metabolism. I have been consulting with Derek for years, and he always gives me great advice as well as the latest findings on nutrition and fitness. The chapter on Sleep is filled with the wisdom from America's "Sleep Doctor," Michael Breus, PhD. I have been astonished to discover how many people suffer from sleep problems, and so I went to my good friend, Dr Breus, to get some answers. In the chapter on Healthy Aging we hear from integrative medical doctor, Bruce Berman, MD, whom I have been consulting with for the last few years. He has given me some excellent advice that has worked for me and may be helpful to you as well. And finally, the chapter on Sexuality is brimming over with sound advice and the latest information from Lou Paget, AASECT. (She is a sex educator—the person whom sex therapists learn from). I keep in touch with Lou on a regular basis, asking her questions that are on the minds of so many women that I speak with. I think that what she has to say may be as helpful to you as it's been to me.

All of these professionals are outstanding in their fields and are known and respected internationally for their knowledge and expertise.

Due to my choices and some unexpected acts of grace, I've defied the norms of society in a way that have made me rethink what the "prime" years of life really are—and it is definitely not all downhill from age 25 or even 40! As I began to think about what it means to truly go through life gracefully, my goal has always been to inspire the younger generation to look forward to *all* of the years that lie ahead because we never know what life is going to bring—the best years of our lives may very well lie in the future.

If there's one thing I know for sure, it's this....It's simply not true that retirement spells the end of the road ---we should continue to explore life, challenge ourselves, and to be open to new ideas. When I look ahead, I see an amazing world filled with infinite possibilities that beckon even as I grow older.

To travel through life gracefully has as much to do with our inner attitude and gratitude toward life as it does with having curiosity and an inquisitive mind. It has to do with seeking ways in which to bring joy and abundance into our own life and spreading them to others. And it has to do with being more interested in others than we are in ourselves. Living a fit, young and vital life is about many things. It encompasses our spiritual and intellectual beings as well as our physical beings. Living an enriched life is the true meaning of living life to its fullest, and if you can do so with grace, all the better.

Different chapters throughout the first half of this book address the fundamentals of being fit, young and vital. They are the foundation for creating What's Next.

By being fit you'll find the energy and stamina to accomplish not only the day-to-day tasks, but you'll also be able to pursue whatever it is that is calling out to you. Have you ever noticed that someone who's fit, strong and healthy has a glow and a confidence that is unmistakable? Let's face it—it's sexy! That kind of glow will draw others to you in a stronger, more positive way than a pretty face ever could, and it definitely will help to open more doors.

Being fit throughout life is one of several ways to enhance your vitality and live a full life with energy and enthusiasm, even when illness or other difficulties strike. Vitality is the key to living well. If youth is a state of body and mind, vitality is a state of being—of your soul. If you radiate vitality, youth will follow. Vitality is reflective of your higher self, and if it runs high within you, you are likely leading a happy, healthy life filled with stimulating friends of all ages, a healthy relationship, and a career or some other life choice that keeps you waking up before the alarm goes off every morning.

Oh my—I do sound like a bit of a Pollyanna, don't I? All this talk about "joy and vitality." What about the bad stuff? Surely that is a part of life that we have all faced and had to deal with, some to horrific degrees. I have had my own challenges, and although I see no point in dwelling on them (because we all have them) I will tell you about a few of them. My parents divorced when I was four, I was sent off to boarding school at the age of seven, (a lonely experience for a young child), and all of my summers were spent with a very difficult and demanding father and stepmother. I never had the security of a loving family in my daily life, and homesickness was something I had to learn to live with.

I survived, however, primarily because I was also blessed with a wonderful mom and stepfather (my Poppy) even though I never felt that I had had enough time with them, and some very good and loving friends. I felt that I was always saying "goodbye," and to this day, can't stand airport sendoffs.

In Part Two of this book you will read how, on the first week of my dream job, I was diagnosed with both cancer and a very serious heart condition. It was decision time—to give up or to persevere. I chose the latter.

So when I write about living life with joy and vitality, what I am really writing about is how do we put the "bad stuff" behind us and emerge strong, healthy and optimistic—ready to live our best lives ever? This is what I discovered:

Vitality is the essence of our souls that helps drive who we are and where we're going. When our vitality levels run high, we can face life's difficult times with courage and confidence. We are always being tested, and when we rise above our challenges and face them, we grow and move on. Vitality brings vigor and passion to everything we do. It's likely that vitality played a role in your accomplishments, because without it, success is almost impossible. A vital person exudes self-confidence and inner beauty. She is strong in mind and purpose. She leads a rich and fulfilling life balanced with loving friends and family, activities and interests, as well as a career (if that's one of her choices), or a position of leadership in her community.

Wisdom, grace, and vitality are characteristics that we use to define people we respect and aspire to emulate. I have lived my life inspired by others with these traits. My mother, as you'll read, was my main inspiration...a talented, intelligent career woman way ahead of her time. She was the essence of class, vitality, wit and humor. Having healthy role models in all areas of our lives allows us to discover through others the qualities and traits that we want to live by, while also allowing us to define what these might mean to us personally. A role model is a guiding force for us to observe and learn from; they do not set the rules, however, because that would be doing us a disservice. Rather, they assist in shaping our thoughts, attitudes, and beliefs. They are there when we have questions, when we falter, and mostly when we succeed. Through these experiences, we can apply what we've learned from our role models and develop our own critical thinking patterns and our own original thoughts. Achieving that is what identifies us as individuals.

I have strived to set my own standards for what I believe lead to a healthy, engaged and joyful life. In this book I'll guide you through my approach to living with joy and vitality, and my wish is that you'll be inspired enough to take action in your own life. Come along while I lead you toward the discovery of your own What's Next!

CHAPTER 2: Body Beautiful

Believe in yourself and all that you are. Know that there is something inside you that is greater than any obstacle.

-— Christian Larson

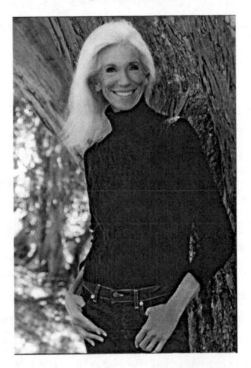

When we think about our bodies, the first thing we ought to remember is that the perception we have of ourselves is often very different from the way others view us. We are our own worst critics! It's interesting, but when we are not loving ourselves, including our bodies, we are subconsciously sending a message to others not to love us as well. Whether verbally or otherwise, disrespecting our bodies damages our self-esteem and causes others to look at us in a less than perfect light.

Over decades, and even centuries, what society has labeled as beautiful has changed drastically. Even today, there are varying degrees of what is seen as beautiful from culture to culture. Some cultures prize bodies that are straight and slim; others value curves and voluptuousness; in actuality, there really isn't one ideal, universal body shape. There are only healthy, well-nourished, beautiful bodies, and ones that are not. This is nothing new.

As a model, (and as a woman) my goal is to present a healthy body and a healthy image of self, not a soulless waif on a runway. I believe that I bring a different attitude to the field of modeling that is much more spiritual and mental than physical. And it works. People are realizing that the perfect body doesn't have to be that of an eighteen year old. It's the attitude that resonates from within that matters. When people ask me about modeling, I tell them that it's about being proud of who I am and projecting that image into the camera lens or on the runway. I believe that real beauty is defined by the way we look at life, by the confidence and wisdom we've acquired along the way, by our life's experiences, and by the joy and love we radiate. Real beauty shines through from the heart and soul. It reflects who we are and where we've been. That is the meaning of beauty. That is aging with grace.

I have had two recent experiences that underscore the truth in this. The first one was a TODAY Show appearance I did in March of 2012. The segment was called Ageless Beauty. I was on the set with Ann Curry and Donny Deutsch, and the topic was how Hollywood and Madison Avenue are beginning to recognize the wisdom and the value of using real looking models in their ads. A 60-year old woman doesn't want to buy wrinkle cream from a 20 year old! And look at some of the recent films that have featured somewhat older women in lead roles—Helen Mirren, Meryl Streep and Sandra Bullock, to name a few.

The other experience I had was just after that show was aired. I was recruited by two international modeling agencies—Silver Models in Paris, and the Ben Barry Agency in Toronto. Ben Barry is known for Diversity in Fashion, and they represent beautiful women of all sizes and ages. Silver Models is an offshoot of Masters Models in Paris, a long established agency, and it came about because of the growing demand for older models.

Let's relate this to photography for a minute. Interestingly enough, the best pictures taken of us are not the ones where our hair is perfect, or where we took shot after shot to get it just right; the best photos of us are the ones where we're emotionally happy, or thinking about someone or something we love when the shutter clicks. This shows us that beauty radiates from how we feel within.

So, why don't we make a habit of presenting ourselves in the best way possible when the camera is not on us? In the moment that the flash is going off, we are aware of the image we are projecting to others—and that should always be an image of self-confidence.

One thing I really want to stress in this book is how to boost your self-confidence and present yourself with pride because the more positive energy you project, the more others see you as a positive, healthy being, and more importantly—the more you become that person. By feeling good about yourself you start to make changes in your self-image and the bodily changes will follow.

With the knowledge and the tools we have available to us, we can change our body to some degree through diet and exercise, and we can change our look with the right fashion choices. But changing our self-image, and levels of self-confidence, isn't as easy.

Body Language Says it All

One of the easiest ways we can begin to project self-confidence is through body language. Becoming aware of our body language, and what it says to others about us, is an essential part of being your most beautiful best self. The next time you're around a group of people, take a mental note of your body language. When you're in a meeting, notice if you are sitting up with confidence, or are you slouching in your seat? Do you cover your mouth when you talk, or are you open and energetic? Do you look down at the floor when speaking with someone or do you look them in the eye with confidence? While body language sends all sorts of messages as to how you feel about those around you, it also sends a message about how you feel about yourself. Not many, if any, people are completely happy with their bodies. The goal is to be happy *within* your body, to accept it, flaws and all, and to project this happiness to the world around you. When you can accomplish this feat, your self-image will soar.

There has been so much research done on the idea of body language that almost everyone is familiar with the concept. So, when we're meeting people, body language is a good place to start. For instance, the way you carry yourself—shoulders back, head high, and chin up, especially while walking—lets people know that you are confident. And believe it or not, confidence without arrogance is sexy!

When we walk, sit or stand with pride, we send that energy out to others. By putting our best foot forward, we camouflage what we believe to be our lesser qualities and project ourselves in a way that others will respond to positively. Looking people in the eye as we offer a warm smile and a firm handshake immediately projects a strong, confident image. This projection is so important because, after all, we only have one chance to make a first impression!

When you think about it, loving your body is really only secondary to loving your inner self. If you have self-love — in other words, if you believe in yourself, respect yourself, and have confidence in yourself — you are going a long way toward loving your body as a part of your whole being. Sure, having a great shape is something we'd all like, but really—when you're with someone, it isn't their shape you're responding to, it's the personality and energy that they exude that attracts you to them. We all have things we don't like about ourselves, but if we let our energy and inner sparkle shine through, if we are genuinely interested in others and care more about them than we do ourselves, then that's what people are going to relate to. I discuss this idea of loving yourself in another chapter, but I think it's important to include it here as well, because it's all tied together. We all need to put less importance on our real or perceived faults and more emphasis on our real selves. In fact, the two most common features that rank high in the polls of attraction are someone's eyes and smile...that should tell us what really matters about a body beautiful!

CHAPTER 3: Come Workout With Me!

If we are creating ourselves all the time, then it is never too late to begin creating the bodies we want instead of the ones we mistakenly assume we are stuck with."

— Deepak Chopra

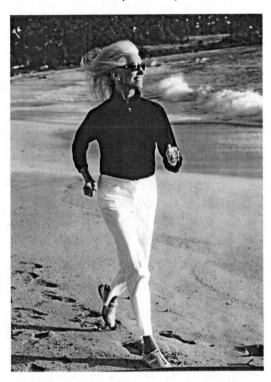

The fundamental benefits of becoming and staying physically fit and active that I wrote about in *Gracefully* have remained constant, and so for those of you who may have missed them before, they bear repeating here. Let me go on to say, however, that there is another extremely important element to the subject of exercise that I have just recently become aware of, and I am eager to share it with you. We will get to that in a moment, but let's go over the basics again first.

As we know, the benefits of exercise have been proven for years. Granted, some of the advice has changed and been tweaked depending on studies, fads, and other factors, but the underlying message is the same: exercise is good for you! We know that being physically fit combats the downfalls of aging and health deterioration. Exercise creates life-loving endorphins that leave us on a natural high. It boosts our metabolism and builds muscles that keep our bones and bodies strong. To me, one of the greatest benefits of staying fit is having the endurance to enjoy life and doing everything I want to do. Without that extra energy, I wouldn't enjoy playing with my grandchildren, walking on the beach with my husband, or rushing off to a modeling assignment or a speaking engagement.

The biggest excuse we hear for not working out is lack of time. There is no one simple answer for building a workout routine or fitness activity into your life, as everyone's schedules and lifestyles vary. The most obvious fact is that you simply *have* to want to do it! That's not to say it won't take a while to grow to enjoy it or to endure the initial muscle soreness. It means that by taking the time to exercise, the health and vitality you will gain from it will be worth it.

> *Physical fitness is not only one of the most important keys to a healthy body; it is the basis of dynamic and creative intellectual activity.*

> John F Kennedy

Getting Started

Let me stress at the outset, that before you begin on any exercise program, it is extremely important that you check with your doctor first. Once you've been given the green light, then you can proceed with whatever form of exercise appeals to you.

One of the healthiest approaches to exercise is "mindful exercise." So what is Mindful Exercise all about? I am quoting Ashley Solomon, Psy.D., She explains it simply and beautifully on her website: www.nourishingthesoul.com: "Mindful Exercise involves being aware of our bodies and minds during physical activity. It means tuning in rather than tuning out, and allowing ourselves to be fully present even in moments of discomfort." *Why would we want to do that?* There are numerous benefits. Consider a few of them:

"Harvard psychologist Ellen Langer and her student found that making women more aware during physical activity resulted in lowering their blood pressure, decreasing their body weight and body fat, and improving waist to hip ratios. The women in the study did not change their behavior; they simply became aware that they were engaging in physical activity.

"Mindful Exercise serves as a great practice of mindfulness in our daily lives. If we exercise daily—whether it's more formally by going to a gym or simply by playing with our children or going for a brisk walk, we have a built in time to practice being more present in our lives. And we know that, like meditation, this practice can lead to decreased depression and anxiety, decreased stress, improved immune functioning, stronger relationships, and better sleep. It's like a Magic Pill!

"Mindful exercise also tunes us into our bodies. If we stay focused and aware of the various points of tension and stress, we can detect problems more quickly and potentially avoid more serious injury.

"Mindful Exercise can make us better athletes. When we're able to tune into the way that our bodies move and flow, our performance improves. To be on top of our game, we have to be operating with intention and focus. In competitive sports, mindfulness gives athletes an edge by increasing perception and reaction time.

"If you're a runner, it may help to supplement your more intense aerobic workouts with a lower-intensity, mindfulness-based practice, such as yoga. A recent study found that even a single session of yoga produced mood-enhancement in participants. Stepping off the elliptical and into a yoga or Pilates class will help you learn to focus your awareness and stay more present as your body moves.

It might be helpful to start by becoming aware of the following:

- Breathing—Notice the rate of your breathing, the feeling as your chest rises and falls, and even the sound.
- Heart Rate—Notice how your heart feels as it pumps blood to the rest of your body.
- Muscle Pangs—Observe all the little twinges, and make sure to stop if the twinges are actually pain.
- Areas of tension—Notice where your body feels tighter and looser. Focus on what it feels like to have your muscles contract and release.
- Joints—Observe the feeling as your body moves at

your joints. Is it smooth? Creaky?

- Thoughts—Notice any thoughts that come into your mind. If they are critical, observe them and come back to your breath.

Just like everything related to mindfulness, mindful exercise takes practice. You're likely to find your mind in all sorts of different places and tied up in all different ways, and that's okay. Stay aware that even by engaging in a few moments of mindfulness per day, you're treating your mind, body, and spirit in a whole new way."

Along with Mindful Exercise is its equally focused partner, Intentional Exercise. Briefly stated, Intentional Exercise is defined by having a specific desired goal and outcome combined with the ability to be intentionally aware and focused on that goal. The best athletes know that Intentional Exercise is made up of three components: understanding which actual exercises will help you to achieve your goal, their required proper form and alignment for best results, and which muscles you will be working.

If your goal is to lose weight, you will want to increase your cardio workouts because this is what burns the calories that will help you lose weight. Add light weights for sculpting because when you couple cardio and strength training, you build muscles, which burn fat. Sculpting your body as you lose weight helps in two ways: 1) it gives you a leaner look as the weight comes off, and 2) muscles burn calories (fat doesn't), so adding muscle through sculpting gives you the extra calorie burning boost needed to expedite weight loss. When the fat comes off, the muscles will readily reveal themselves. In order to design the right program for you, I encourage you to find a personal trainer that you can work with to achieve your goals. Many gyms provide new members with a free fitness analysis, which will help get you off to the right start.

Habits, once formed, can be difficult to break, and exercise is one good habit to develop. Have you ever heard the old adage that if you do something every day for twenty-one days, it becomes a habit? I think it's true!

What inspires you to jump out of bed in the morning? The aroma of coffee brewing in your kitchen? Or is it the thought of going to the gym or out for a walk or run? No matter what form it takes, when exercise influences your desire to leap out of bed and get going, you can be certain that you're living a vital life. You know that you'll feel alive and vibrant by the time you finish that run, lifting weights, swimming, yoga, or whatever your physical passion happens to be. If you've never caught the exercise bug, know that it can be contagious at any age. In fact, I've heard of many people who start jogging or running in their sixties or seventies. These inspirational people are highly regarded for their willingness to begin a new endeavor, especially a challenging one. Many people enter running races and revel in how much younger they feel coming down the home stretch with people half their age. Even if they walk over the finish line, their accomplishment is a worthy one. Their stories are written up in the papers. They're interviewed as a lifestyle or sports story. No matter where you see these newfound athletes, note the large smiles on their faces. Those smiles are there because they feel alive and they have discovered one of the secrets to capturing youth. Their doctor visits often report reduced cholesterol and lower blood pressure. Family members note the athlete's heightened moods. Years drop off their faces, and just being around these people leaves you feeling invigorated. It is contagious. Go to any track early in the morning, and I'll bet you'll see some newly indoctrinated walkers and joggers who have some years behind them. I clink my water bottle to theirs.

Because exercise comes in so many forms and has so many venues, it often isn't about keeping weight down or putting muscle on; it provides many emotional, mental and social advantages. Whether you take part in golf, tennis, yoga, swimming, softball, or any other sport, you've likely met some wonderful people and have developed solid friendships through these events and related activities. For example, many golf tournaments or marathons entail volunteerism and philanthropy. The sense of community engendered by these events is remarkable and beneficial to everyone involved.

If there's one theme that has strongly developed in our society, it's the acceptance that no matter what stage or age you're at in life, when you begin a workout routine or take up a sport, it's always accepted and encouraged by others who are already doing it. Options such as hiring a personal trainer for a one-on-one introduction to a routine, or joining a beginners running group or yoga class, all work to satisfy anyone's comfort level for getting started.

Some people may prefer to workout in the privacy of their homes, or they may not have access to a gym. Some may even be confined to their homes for health reasons; however, if a gym membership or your local senior center is an option for you, membership can offer an abundance of opportunities besides treadmills or elliptical trainers. There is often a variety of classes available ranging from beginning to advanced levels.

When looking into the different classes offered at your gym, note that there are usually different instructors for each class, and it's worth trying a few of them if your schedule permits. Finding the right instructor can make a big difference in how much you enjoy the class! Bring a full water bottle and wear appropriate clothing. One of the biggest advantages of falling into a routine of going to a class is meeting and bonding with the other regulars over sweat. Many friendships have been formed within gym walls. And believe me, they will notice if you miss a class!

Pilates and Yoga

Pilates and yoga classes are two choices that have people sitting, stretching and performing moves and stances they would normally never think of doing, and they love it! These classes are invigorating and you'd be hard pressed to find a more suitable workout for a body to age gracefully, but also be prepared to laugh at yourself if you're a beginner. Everyone goes through that awkward stage of figuring out the names positions, let alone the actual physicality of them. It's a plight that is overcome with time if you stick to it! And the benefits are many. The low impact movements are important for seniors and those who can't endure high impact. The slow movements allow for building a strong mental connection to each position and the transition between positions, allowing you to feel connected in body, mind, and even soul. The physical benefits of these classes will also keep your muscles long and supple and graceful.

The primary concept with Pilates, yoga and other exercise methodologies is the coordination of breath and movement. Not only do these classes help to keep your circulatory system and other systems healthy, but Yoga, in particular, through the ages, has always focused on the breath. Although Joseph Pilates worked a great deal with veterans returning from war, his ideas evolved and became very popular with dancers, especially in New York City. His students became the teachers that have carried the Pilates tradition forward and helped develop its current popularity. Joseph Pilates designed many exercises in order to strengthen and bring the body into balance, and to lengthen and strengthen the muscles.

Having an instructor to guide you through the class is not only safer, but most likely there are others in the class at your level from whom you can learn. A good, certified instructor will make the class enjoyable, and hopefully you'll go back time and time again. One such instructor is Olava Menczkowska. Olava strives to provide a healthy, warm, safe environment for her clients. As an experienced Pilates and dance instructor, she encourages fluid and graceful movement in her classes.

Olava has been in the movement field for over thirty years and throughout that time she has naturally seen changes in the workouts, the clients, and the age groups of those involving themselves in her programs. "The paradigm of exercise has shifted, and I certainly see that in my own experience over the past ten, twenty, and thirty years. The next wave, or the wave we seem to be in now, is where we're formulating a composite of those very same principles of breath and movement blended with other movement and dance forms to strike a chord of health, well-being and physical functionality for today's more physically inactive world.

In reflecting on her clients, Olava said, "I have a lot of elderly people that I absolutely adore. The ages range from ten to ninety years old in my classes." These are clients who return week after week, support one another, and as a community, bond over stretching and feeling revitalized, literally to their core.

The ultimate goal for everyone taking a class in Pilates or yoga is to find their body in balance. Olava tells her clients to, "Find your own music. Find your own breath. Find those and there is the correlation between breath and music."

The Benefits of Yoga and Pilates

The benefits of all the stretching, posturing, and breathing properly are both visible and invisible. On the exterior, you'll begin to see definition and tone that you didn't have before. Your face will be aglow as you head out the door for the rest of your day. On the invisible side, the benefits to your inner body are paramount. All of the systems of your body–from your circulatory system to your nervous system to systems we don't even know about can benefit from the body realignment techniques of yoga and Pilates.

In some sense, Pilates and yoga "unbunches" you. A workout will leave you feeling fresh and untangled. In no time, you'll find yourself sitting up straighter and walking taller due to the lengthening and toning of muscles. The beauty of workouts such as these is that they go in tandem with other workouts or activities that you're involved in. If it's the only exercise you do, that's great, but if you are a cross trainer, you'll soon notice a positive difference in your other endeavors. Gaining the fluidity that the stretching and breathing bring to you, you'll function much better in all that you do.

If a class is intimidating, but the idea tantalizing, try a yoga or Pilates DVD. There are also several options available. Masters such as Rodney Yee has several good yoga DVDs, especially for beginners, as does Peggy Cappy. Her DVD, "Yoga: For the Rest of Us and More" is geared toward beginners.

Spinning and Body Pump

For a higher energy workout, spinning (indoor cycling) is a favorite for many gym goers. The low impact makes it easier on the body, but make sure to check your bike's settings with the instructor before starting. The great thing about spinning is that while the instructors provide guidance throughout the class, you can go at your own pace to an extent. Not only does it work your legs and raise your heart rate, some instructors incorporate upper body movements such as little pushups into their routine. The upbeat music will keep you going, and be prepared to sweat! Even the beginning classes will give you a hard workout. An important tip: wear cycling shorts (padded for comfort!), and as with any aerobic class, bring a water bottle.

Body Pump is a popular class among those who want to integrate some weight training with aerobic activity. This, too, is guided by the instructor and the amount of weight you use depends on your desire and ability. Wearing comfortable clothes, especially those that allow sweat to wick away from your body, is suggested. The high energy of this class will tone muscles and burn fat in one class. Now that's a great combination!

No matter what class you take, I recommend talking to the instructors prior to class to find out as much as you can and about what to expect. A personal trainer might be able to give you some guidance as well. In general, classes run 45 minutes to an hour or more and, if applicable, they will note if it's a beginner or advanced class. Check their schedule.

Weight Training

If you want to expand your workout horizons and venture into weight training, I strongly urge you to enlist with a knowledgeable, certified and experienced personal trainer—but again, check with your doctor first.

The Great Outdoors

The examples described so far in this chapter are geared toward indoor workouts. For outdoor enthusiasts, there are the traditional activities such as golf, tennis, running, cycling, hiking, kayaking, skiing, and several others, which vary in intensity, price, simplicity, and availability. Three of my daughters, Darcy, Anne and Heather, are all cyclists who engage in the sport for very different reasons. Darcy competes, Heather uses it as a muse for her writing, and Anne enjoys casual mountain biking with friends. They all have different motivations, yet they all benefit from the same activity.

Sports like swimming, naturally, can be done inside or out depending on the season. Gyms with swimming pools often have water aerobic classes available. Or, local colleges and city pools may be available. As recommended in the "Learn Something New" chapter, there are websites such as www.meetup.com that you can look into for joining other outdoor sporting enthusiasts. This is especially helpful if you're not only new to a sport but new to an area and want to meet people while also having the opportunity to be outdoors and exercising!

The beautiful thing about exercise is that it doesn't have to be routine or forced. The options are endless in so many ways: availability, simplicity, cost, equipment, team or group vs. individual, and there are certified instructors and trainers—the list goes on and on. If you can find your niche in the workout world, you'll be certain to open new doors to a physically healthier and happier future.

As an early riser, my choice to exercise at home first thing in the morning fits well into my daily routine. Others find it easier to join a gym or work out with friends, or they may prefer to do their workouts in the evening. No matter when or where, the important thing is creating the habit, and let me stress again, seeking the advice of a doctor and a personal trainer before starting is, as always, recommended.

The ideal way to start any program is to start with small, achievable goals and to build up to a full routine. The best of intentions, as we know from New Year's resolutions, fail when you take on more than you can handle at any one time. Examine your daily and weekly routine and plug in a planned time for exercise. Fix that time on your calendar the same way you would a doctor's appointment, business meeting, or attendance at an event with your child or grandchild. If you can't make a trip to the gym to spend an hour on the treadmill, plan a long, brisk walk as you go about your day. Make your time work efficiently and be realistic about how you're going to make exercise an ongoing part of your life.

There is a great quote by Gloria Steinman. Loosely stated, apparently someone remarked to Ms. Steinman that she did not look fifty, to which Steinman answered, "My dear this *is* what fifty looks like." Finding a healthy and safe way to mesh exercise into your schedule allows you to enjoy your body well into old age. Whether with friends, in a class, or on your own, it's an essential aspect to Creating What's Next—Gracefully!

CHAPTER 4: The Benefits of Proper Nutrition Advice from a Nutritionist

Our bodies are our gardens – our wills are our gardeners.

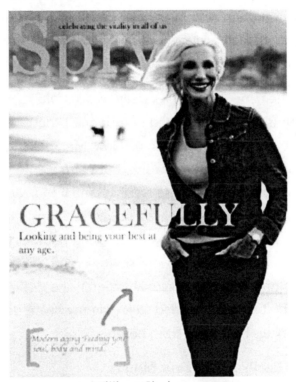

— William Shakespeare

We gain so much wisdom as we move into our mid-life years, and one of the key areas where this truism is so blatantly clear is when it comes to nutrition. When I was younger I rarely gave any thought to what I was going to eat that day. If I was in the mood for a hamburger—pasta—chicken—fish—a salad—Red Devil cake! Well sure, why not? Did eating properly make a difference in how I felt? Was my energy higher on a healthy diet than when I was negligent about it? I never noticed. In your twenties and thirties, you rarely pay attention to those things. You are too consumed with Living! But as I got older, and particularly as I took on more and more responsibilities, first as a busy mom and then as a career woman, all of a sudden nutrition started to take on a very important role in my life. I noticed a big difference in my stamina and all around health when I book better care of myself nutritionally.

In 2003 when my modeling career was unfolding, I consulted Derek Johnson, a renowned nutrition expert and holistic nutritionist and the cofounder of New Metabolism. I not only wanted to ensure my future health, but I also wanted to increase my energy level. Both of these were essential to keeping up with the demands of my position as public relations manager at a world-famous golf resort and an increasing number of modeling assignments. Johnson's proven outlook and philosophies on nutrition, along with the personal program he designed for me, provided the balance I needed to juggle my hectic schedule and the many meals I eat away from home.

What You Really Put in Your Mouth

What follows is how I worked with a personal nutritionist and how you can too—even if you don't have one in your area and need to do it remotely (as I did). To those of you who have read my earlier book, *Gracefully—Looking and Being Your Best at Any Age*, this will be familiar territory, but it is one (of those core elements) that I absolutely felt was worth repeating because the principals and good information I'm about to share with you are just as true today as they were five years ago.

Even if you believe you eat a healthy diet, working with an established nutritionist will open your eyes to so much more than just what you put in your mouth. As a foundation for all of his clients' programs Johnson uses a nutritional analysis that includes personal and family histories, a physical activity profile, a dietary assessment, segmental body fat testing, and integrative lab tests. While much of the dietary advice Johnson provides is universal, all of his clients have their own body chemistry makeup, which he looks at when determining what's missing from their diets. A personalized program based on the results of his analysis leads to an optimum eating plan for each person's body and lifestyle.

I was impressed with his approach because it focuses on two vital areas that unhealthy people often neglect—proper digestion and sleep requirements. (See next chapter for Tips for Getting a Good Night's Sleep). Working toward proper digestion made sense to me, but I wouldn't have thought that sleep mattered as much as it does when it comes to nutrition. For these reasons and many more, Johnson opposes fad diets that produce short-term, unsustainable results, especially because these diets go against the two core requirements of adequate digestion and sleep. What I love about his approach is that he looks at the body image as a whole, as well as how his clients feel about themselves emotionally and physically.

"Simple Rules to Live By for a Healthy Life:" (see sidebar) are a great place for anyone to start. These lists are taped to my bathroom mirror as a reminder of the simple daily steps I can take toward being healthier. They have now become habits, just like brushing my teeth. While not complicated, the plan that Johnson devised for me changes as my schedule and routine change, such as when I'm traveling or have a modeling assignment on the horizon. For instance, he suggested that I eat more protein and fewer carbs for a few days before a modeling assignment or a big social engagement so I don't get the bloated-belly feeling that can kick in by four o'clock. I've also found that the well-known mantra of a big healthy breakfast, a balanced lunch, and a light dinner early in the evening works wonders for keeping my stomach flat and knocking off a couple of pounds for that all-important occasion.

My positive approach to life meshed well with Johnson's conviction that you have to become healthy to lose weight. In my case it was a matter of building muscle tissue, which can add weight to an already slight frame. So, although weight loss wasn't an issue for me, finding energy through my diet and adding muscle tone were critical. There are several body types, and being thin doesn't necessarily mean you're healthier than someone who needs to shed some weight. Also, you need to redefine *weight* as "body fat" rather than the number you read on the scale. Muscle tissue and body fat are what matter, and most women do not have enough muscle. It's about your clothing size, not the number on the scale. In regards to the philosophy of being healthy to lose weight, Johnson adds, "You have to be healthy for the body to maintain its ideal weight; you cannot force it to do so from dieting."

The skinny is that many underweight people are starved for crucial nutrients, meaning they are technically unhealthy. "In actuality, many thin people feel much worse than overweight people, but you would never know it from their looks," he explains. "The body is malnourished, which means it starts to use muscle for energy. This is what puts women at more risk for osteopenia, the precursor of osteoporosis. Each person's body knows exactly where its healthy weight is, and it's our job to fuel the body properly so that it can do the rest. By eating the right foods each day, it will build and maintain the right amount of muscle and keep off any unwanted body fat."

Like exercise, a sensible, balanced diet should become a habit, which is why fad programs don't work. Any limited diet may take weight off initially but those diets are not healthy in the long run and are impossible to stick to—they are technically designed to fail. It has been proven over and over that you need a balance of protein, carbohydrates, and fats. So go for the long haul. While you may lose weight at a slower pace, it will stay off and you'll feel much better.

Need more reasons to eat well? How about anti-aging: What usually comes to mind when you think of looking younger: Probably hair color, shampoos, skin care formulas and creams, or supplements. Johnson notes, "Trying to just look healthy on the outside isn't as important as becoming healthy on the inside. The answer once again is proper sleep and digestion. You cannot trick the body long term; that only works with short-term things like makeup and eye creams. But we have to remember to treat the cause, not the symptom. For example, someone may have a stomachache, bloating, or gas several times a week, so we commonly identify things like food allergies from simple blood test that might be the cause of these symptoms. Remember, if you're not healthy from the beginning, your body isn't going to maintain the results you desire. This goes for all types of people, from stay-at-home moms to professional athletes."

Digestion, Johnson admits, is not a "cool" thing to talk about, but even if you're eating well and taking supplements, if you're not taking in the right nutrients, your daily function is thrown off. "There's a laundry list of things your body must have to stay alive—pretty skin and nails are at the bottom of the list. In terms of anti-aging the body's largest organ is the skin, and it tells everything about us—it comes back to digesting and absorbing foods properly."

When I first met with Johnson, he asked me two basic questions: what foods I liked and how I felt throughout the day. He said, "Get your body in tune as much as you can through food, because without that, it's an uphill battle." These words still resonate with me.

With the children grown and gone, baby boomers finally have the chance to take better care of themselves. It's never too late to start focusing on your health, even if you haven't done so before. Diets in the United States tend to be acidic, and acidic bodies are a sickness magnet. We all know about heart disease and diabetes. "You pay for things later in life because the body has a funny way of letting you know eventually that you didn't take care of it. The better the body functions, the better it's going to recover and repair," Johnson reminds his clients. "Your body is constantly changing. It adapts to both good and bad environments alike. Yet it doesn't always tell you you're being unhealthy, which is why heart disease is the number-one killer in women. A few of the fundamental rules about nutrition are fact. It's unfortunate that people take the basic concepts of nutrition and try to make up their own rules..... Over time, everything we eat has a direct effect on our health, and that's a fundamental fact that can't be manipulated."

As I discussed in Chapter 3, I didn't incorporate a regular workout routine into my schedule until later in life. Incidentally, this is one of Johnson's requirements—that each client create a workout routine that integrates resistance training. "To build muscle tone, it's important to do resistance training, especially for clients who aren't that mobile and can't move around due to a bad hip," he notes. "There are exercises they can do if they're shown how to do them properly."

Johnson discusses osteoporosis with clients as young as their thirties and forties and with thinner clients because they often aren't getting the proper nutritional absorption that comes from a lack of muscle tissue. He loves the idea of getting in a swimming pool with floaties for resistance training, saying that it's "often better than any medicine they can take."

Winning the anti-aging war doesn't happen overnight, but it is truly amazing what the body can do and recover from once you come face-to-face with what food is and how it works inside your body. When you're eating foods that work well for you, you don't have to worry about digesting. Coupled with a good night's sleep, that eating well can take years off your looks and add them to your life.

Valerie's Nutrition Program

I've always had a sweet tooth, and my personal nutritional program revolves around curbing my cookie cravings. Since the brain runs on glucose, you create an imbalance when you eat a lot of sugar; the brain tries to catch up and you end up in a constant flux of too much sugar or not enough. Derek taught me that by increasing the protein and "good" carbohydrates in my diet and having fruit for a snack, I could decrease my cookie cravings. It was difficult at first, but I soon found out that he was right. The discovery of a cracker (carried by Whole Foods) that is both gluten-free and low in sugar really helped. You can spread a thin layer of almond or peanut butter on a few of these crackers and feel just as satisfied as you would have if you'd eaten an oatmeal raisin cookie! Check your health food store or grocery store for cookies that don't contain any of the "bad" ingredients you want to avoid and that are still tasty—just as good as their more fattening counterparts. When I want to treat myself to a cookie, I'll reach for one or two of these.

One item Johnson removed from my diet was soy protein powder, substituting whey protein powder instead. He explained to me that most soy is not a desirable form of protein for many reasons, one being that it is almost all genetically modified or GMO,. "Soy is fine if it's an old-fashioned fermented soy product such as tempeh and natto, all of which can be incorporated into any type of lifestyle. Using soy milk, soy protein powder, and soy burgers—things we've marketed and used misleading and false information about in the United States—can reduce the absorption of many important nutrients, not to mention it can have a direct effect on your body's hormones," he notes. "Remember, the United States is one of the unhealthiest nations in the world, and one of the most overweight, too. There is solid evidence linking soy to cognitive decline, reproductive disorders, and immune system breakdowns. Whey protein is so much better. It is a great idea if you can get grass fed Whey! It's great for smoothies and is perfect for a post-workout drink. Make sure to add glutamine to the protein shake, which is important for the lining of the stomach and helps build mass for muscle tissue." My personal favorite is to whip up a shake of protein powder, orange-flavored Emergen-C, four ounces of fresh squeezed orange juice, and two ounces of cran-raspberry juice. For a meal on the run, I'll pop this in a thermos, grab a protein bar, and I head out the door. Another quick favorite for breakfast when I'm in a hurry is to have a slice of multi-grain whole wheat bread from the bakery, spread with crunchy almond butter and a little marmalade—along with one of these protein drinks. Filling and nutritious!

Together, Johnson and I added several foods to my diet, including whole eggs, more vegetables, fish, tuna, fruits (berries are best), peanut and almond butter, kidney and black beans, chicken, turkey, rice crackers, hummus, leafy dark green salads, pita or gluten-free cinnamon raison bread (just because I love anything cinnamon raisin, and it's a better choice than cookies), real fruit jams, and goat cheese. Integrating Johnson's plan with my workouts has helped me build muscle, retain energy, and get the stamina and kick I need for a long day of modeling shoots or speaking engagements.

Nutrition and eating right needn't be daunting. There are ample resources available online, in magazines, books, and television shows in addition to doctors and professional nutritionists. The trick is learning how to weed through the data to find the nuggets you need. Keep away from fads and trendy diets because they often result in more damage than benefit. Prepare your grocery list at home by looking through your refrigerator and pantry—are there enough fruits, vegetables, and grains? Glance through a yummy, nutritious website like www.epicurean.com or a cookbook for appealing recipes and jot down the needed ingredients. Many recipes these days provide nutritional data—something they didn't do when I was a young mother. If you can help it, never go to the grocery store when you're hungry, which makes impulse buying irresistible. Prepare your list and then stick to it.

Old habits are easier to break when they're replaced with a new, desirable habit. What do you have to lose? A few pounds? And what you'll gain will reward you tenfold.

From Derek Johnson, New Metabolism

5 RULES:

1- Eat breakfast or a snack within the first 45-60 min of waking.

2- Never eat a starchy carb by itself, always add a fat or protein. (ex: ½ apple with 1tbsp pb)

3- Eat 3 meals and a snack per day, dinner is the smallest

4- Drink 64-80oz of water per day (on non-workout day), only small amounts with meals. Rehydrate with a glass upon waking.

5- Get 7-8 hours of solid sleep each night.

NEW METABOLISM TIPS:

1- Never go longer than 5 hours without eating.

2- Ideally, eat dinner by 7:00 p.m.

3- Take at least one 15-minute break outside during work.

4- Choose unprocessed carbs or ones that come from the ground (ex: rice, yams, sweet potatoes, beans)

5- Limit your portions and eat slowly while seated.

I am often asked, "What do you eat on a typical day?"

I try to include protein and complex carbohydrates with every meal. I think I'm blessed with a good metabolism to begin with and also by not having a terribly large appetite. I don't care for rich foods or a lot of sweets (although I love cookies and do indulge in those—but in moderation!) There is a special brand that Whole Foods carries that doesn't have hydrogenated oils or high fructose corn syrup and tastes delicious.

For breakfast I usually have ½ grapefruit, 2 scrambled eggs with a piece of gluten-free Ezekiel cinnamon raisin toast, and coffee. Steel cut oatmeal is another good choice.

Lunch might be a sliced turkey or tuna sandwich on toasted whole grain bread, or low-fat yogurt with granola and dried cranberries. And dinner is frequently either something like grilled chicken or fish, vegetables and a salad, or a homemade soup with beans, spinach, tomatoes, and ground beef or turkey. I often get hungry around 4 in the afternoon and will whip up a whey protein shake, which I blend with orange and cran-raspberry juices and a packet of Super Orange Emergen-C. (See above— Johnson's advice about whey protein powder with my own recipe for a protein drink).

Another favorite snack—or even breakfast choice—might be the protein smoothie with a slice of toasted multi-grain bread from the bakery with crunchy almond butter and a bit of orange marmalade. High energy—healthy protein and complex carbohydrates, and it sticks with you throughout a busy morning!

I am not an angel, however, and when I go out I pretty much have whatever I like, including a glass of wine and dessert. I don't believe in sacrificing the pleasures of all the wonderful foods that are out there, but I do believe in moderation.

So there you have it... All of the tried and true information on nutrition that I have acquired over the years, and believe me, it works. If I am tired and dragging, there is nothing like a small healthy snack or meal to revitalize me. It makes a significant difference.

CHAPTER 5: Advice From
The Sleep Doctor

It is a common experience that a problem difficult at night is resolved in the morning after the committee of sleep has worked on it.

— John Steinbeck

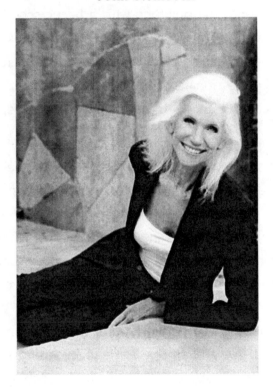

𝒟uring the fifteen years when I was working at Pebble Beach, there were many evenings when I entertained travel writers, celebrities, or producers at one of the several famous restaurants the Resorts have to offer. Things haven't changed much since then, only now on any given evening I may be traveling to give a speech somewhere or off on a modeling assignment. Besides the challenge of eating healthy while dining out, late dinners result in late nights and my sleep suffers as a result. Furthermore, it has seriously come to my attention that I am not alone in sometimes having difficulties in getting a good night's sleep. The more I meet and talk with other people, the more prevalent this problem seems to be.

Of course, I'm not the only one with a hectic schedule. Both Dr. Breus' (www.thesleepdocor.com) and Derek Johnson's (www.newmetabolism.com) diverse client lists include athletes, celebrities, professionals, and full-time parents. Our hectic schedules can fill us with adrenaline, and sleep can be a challenge.

The ideal is seven to eight hours sleep—the key being to obtain at least six hours of uninterrupted sleep. Each person's body requires varying amounts within these guidelines. A lot of people don't realize what's happening to their bodies when they wake up in the middle of the night to use the bathroom or get a drink of water. As Johnson explains, "Our bodies are a chemistry lab, not a bank account. When we interrupt sleep patterns, the process of healing the damage done from the previous day is self-defeating. We add to the damage by losing sleep and we lose out on critical healing that comes from reaching the levels of sleep cycles. "Working on getting solid sleep first is important, and it's never too late to start getting quality sleep," states Johnson. "Staying asleep to get through the sleep cycles, creating that consistency, means you don't want to wake up and restart during the night, or in the morning you'll wake up groggy. Sleep is where we repair from a day's activity. Exercise and activity put us in the red, and the more we stay in the deficit, the more damage we cause. Injuries are more likely to occur then."

Dr. Michael Breus, Phd

Not long ago I had the great honor of being invited to be a presenter at CARP, the Canadian Association of Retired People, in Toronto. At that prestigious conference I was fortunate to meet Dr. Michael Breus, PhD, a popular sleep authority sometimes referred to as "The Sleep Doctor." Michael has graced many TV shows, including numerous appearances on Oprah, Dr. Oz, CNN, Katie and others. He is the author of *BEAUTY SLEEP: Look Younger, Lose Weight, and Feel Great Through Better Sleep.*

As the subject of sleep gains greater momentum in our sleep-deprived society, Dr. Breus has become a widely recognized leader in this highly evolving field. I had no idea how many people have problems with simply getting a good night's sleep until I started giving speeches and found it to be such a prevalent problem. After I speak, whenever possible, I like to open the floor to Q&A, and I was astonished at how often the subject of sleep was brought up. When I consulted with Dr. Breus about this, he gave me lots of good advice and information, most of which I have followed myself and have found to be very helpful. For more information, I recommend that you take a look at Dr. Brues' website www.thesleepdoctor.com. He is the Sleep Expert for WebMD Health, a leading Internet site for health-related information, and you can also find him on The Huffington Post and Psychology Today discussing topics from mattress choice to sleep apnea.

I would like to pass along some very valuable scientific information Michael gave to me on the value of sleep. (You will note that he and Derek Johnson are in agreement on this subject). This is what I learned from Michael:

Benefits of Sleep: Sleep Stages and the Science of Sleep

Sleep is a significant health concern that is just as important as nutrition, exercise and stress management. There are many benefits of sleep, as our bodies heal and recuperate from the wear and tear of our day while we sleep at night.

Getting good, restorative sleep, however, is not just a matter of hitting the pillow at night and waking up in the morning. Regulated by your body clock, your nighttime journey consists of sleep cycles divided into specific sleep stages, all of which are vital for your body and mind. Accordingly, understanding the benefits of sleep cycles and stages can help you get a better night's sleep.

Understanding the Sleep Cycle Stages

There are several different stages of sleep, and each one plays a different part in preparing your mind and body for the following day. There are two main types of sleep:

- Non-REM Sleep (NREM Sleep)
- REM Sleep (Rapid Eye Movement)

    Non-REM sleep consists of four stages of sleep, and each stage is deeper than the previous one. The four cumulative stages of Non-REM sleep are as follows:

- Stage 1 (Transition to sleep)—The first stage of Non-REM sleep, stage 1 lasts about five minutes, where the eyes move slowly under the eyelids and muscle activity slows down. People in this sleep stage are easily awoken. This stage will make up about 5% of the night.

- Stage 2 (Light sleep)—The first stage of true sleep, stage 2 lasts from 10 to 25 minutes per sleep cycle, where heart rate slows, eye movement stops and body temperature decreases. This stage will make up about 50% of the night.

- Stage 3 (Deep sleep)—It is difficult to wake a person in this stage of sleep, where you may feel groggy and disoriented for several minutes upon awakening. This stage (in combination with stage 4) will make up about 25% of the night.

- Stage 4 (More intense deep sleep)—The deepest stage of sleep, stage 4 restores physical energy while blood flow is directed away from the brain and towards the muscles. Brain waves in this stage of sleep are extremely slow.

REM (Rapid Eye Movement) Sleep

Your eyes actually move back and forth during REM sleep, and this is the type of sleep when you do the most active dreaming. REM sleep, or dream sleep, begins about 70 to 90 minutes after you fall asleep. Heart rate and blood pressure increase while breathing becomes shallow, and the arm and leg muscles become paralyzed. This stage represents about 25% of the night.

Beauty Sleep

One of the benefits of sleep is the generation and rejuvenation of skin cells. While asleep, the skin makes new cells twice as fast as it does during our waking hours. Several studies have found that sleep-deprived people have lower levels of a specific growth hormone that the skin needs quality sleep to repair environmental damage acquired during the day. Without it, wrinkles and slackness may result, which is why we have come to call our nighttime rest -"beauty sleep." Notice how revitalized you look even after a refreshing nap! The difference really is noticeable.

Sleep Cycle Disruption

The benefits of sleep may diminish, however, if the sleep cycle is disrupted. Sleep cycle disruption caused by loud noise, excess light or other problems accumulated over time can lead to sleep deprivation.

Sleep Deprivation—Illness and Insulin Resistance

Timi Gustafson, RD, reports in her blog for the Seattle Post Intelligencer, that clinical studies have shown that sleep deprivation can be a contributing factor to a number of lifestyle-related illnesses—among them are obesity, diabetes, hypertension and heart disease. Without proper rest, the brain also works harder but less effectively.

Cortisol

Gustafson also reports that sleeplessness can lead to imbalances in the release of stress hormones, such as cortisol. Potential consequences of cortisol imbalance include:

• Weakening of the immune system
• Risk of a variety of chronic illnesses
• Psychological effects such as memory loss, mood swings and depression

Sleeping for Health and Quality of Life

There is compelling evidence that a healthy sleep routine can contribute greatly to one's physical and mental well-being as well as their overall quality of life. Sufficient sleep ranks among the best defense mechanisms we have to stay healthy and handle our stress. In short, when we get enough nourishing sleep, we are more likely to stay healthy and well all around.

If you are suffering from a sleep problem and looking for additional tips on the benefits of sleep, consult with a doctor or visit a sleep center for diagnosis and treatment.

Sleep problems may contribute to cognitive decline

A group of studies, all conducted independently, have reached a similar sobering conclusion: sleep problems—including several common sleep difficulties faced by millions of people on a regular basis—may, over time, lead to cognitive impairment and even dementia. Sleep deprivation, oversleeping, daytime tiredness, and sleep-disordered breathing—may play a significant role in cognitive decline as we age.

To investigate the relationship between sleep and cognitive decline, researchers examined data from 15,263 women, all of whom were 70 years or older at the time of the first cognitive assessment. Researchers found that sleeping too little and sleeping too much were both associated with cognitive decline over time:

- Women who slept 5 hours a day or less had lower average cognitive scores than women who slept 7

47

hours per day

- Women who slept more than 9 hours had lower average scores than women who slept 7 hours per day
- Women whose sleep duration changed by more than 2 hours—up or down—had lower cognitive assessment scores than women whose daily sleep patterns did not change significantly

A study led by scientists at University of California San Francisco, also examined the relationship between cognitive function and sleep disorders among older women. The results of this study showed a connection between disrupted sleep—especially sleep-disordered breathing—and diminished cognitive function:

- Women with sleep-disordered breathing were more than two times as likely to show evidence of dementia than women without sleep-disordered breathing
- Women who showed signs of disrupted sleep cycles were also more likely to demonstrate cognitive problems and dementia.
- Total sleep time was not associated with cognitive decline among these women. However, women who experienced greater periods of nighttime wakefulness scored lower on their cognitive function tests.

There is more work to be done to establish a causal link between disrupted sleep and cognitive decline. We're still a long way from a real understanding about just how sleep affects cognitive function over the course of a lifetime, and how lack of sleep may contribute to the onset of dementia or other conditions involving cognitive impairment and decline. But such unanimity among the results of no fewer than four separate studies certainly lends credibility to the findings.

The Importance Of Diet And Getting A Good Night's Sleep

In conclusion, I want to add some very important tips about what a difference our diet makes in how we sleep. This is information that we can all benefit from. Again—my thanks to Dr. Breus:

Are you having trouble sleeping? Are your everyday actions normal? Are you getting enough sleep?

If everything in life seems to be running smoothly except for the fact that you cannot get a good night's rest, it may be due to poor diet or the wrong bedtime snacks.

Your daily diet and what you eat before bed does in fact effect how you sleep. Some foods help your sleep habits and others negatively affect it. Foods that are generally good for a full night's sleep contain tryptophan that is a precursor to serotonin and melatonin that help you relax. Spicy foods, stimulants, high-fat meals and overeating may contribute to a poor night's sleep. Some people don't know how much your dinner or what you eat before bed can effect how well you sleep.

What foods contain tryptophan or induce serotonin and

melatonin? Here are 10 foods that are helpful for a good night's sleep:

1. Bananas -- Bananas contain magnesium, a muscle relaxant.

2. Chamomile tea -- Chamomile has a mild calming effect and makes it an excellent natural antidote for restless minds and bodies.

3. Honey -- Drizzle a little in your warm milk or herb tea. A large amount of sugar is stimulating but only a little glucose tells your brain to turn off orexin.

5. Potatoes -- A small baked potato is good for your gastrointestinal tract as it clears away acids that can interfere with yawn-inducing tryptophan. You can also mash the potato with warm milk, speeding up the falling-asleep process.

6. Oatmeal -- Oats are a rich source of sleep-inviting melatonin, and with a small bowl of warm cereal with a splash of maple syrup, you'll be ready for bed in no time.

7. Almonds -- A handful of these healthy nuts will have you snoozing because they contain both tryptophan and dose of muscle-relaxing magnesium.

8. Flaxseeds -- Try sprinkling 2 tablespoons of these little seeds on your bedtime oatmeal. They're rich in omega-3 fatty acids which are a natural mood lifter.

9. Whole-wheat bread -- A slice of toast will release insulin, it helps tryptophan get to your brain, which is then converted to serotonin and sends your body the message that it is time to sleep.

10. Tart cherries—They have the largest source of plant based Melatonin of any plant! There are studies showing that drinking this juice can help with sleep.

Avoid unhealthy foods before bed, keep a balanced diet that includes dairy, whole grains and fruits and you should sleep just fine.

What are some of the benefits of getting a good night's sleep?

- Sleep is just as important as nutrition, exercise and stress management
- Heal and recuperate from the wear and tear of the day
- Regeneration and rejuvenation of skin cells to repair environmental damage and produce new skin cells

Once skin cell replacement falls behind, wrinkles and slackness result. Hence the term, "Beauty Sleep!"

What are some of the dangers of not getting a good night's sleep?

- Sleep deprivation can contribute to obesity, diabetes, hypertension and heart disease
- Without proper rest, we don't think as clearly
- Imbalance of stress hormones such as Cortisol
- Weakening of the immune system
- Risk of a variety of chronic illnesses
- Memory loss, mood swings and depression

Tips On Getting A Good Night's Sleep

- Keep a constant sleep schedule
- Eliminate caffeine by 2 PM

- Stop drinking alcohol 3 hours before lights out. This allows you to metabolize the alcohol you had at dinner
- Your daily diet and what you eat before bed does, in fact, effect how you sleep
- Exercise daily, but try to limit it to not fewer than 4 hours before bedtime
- Get 15 min of sunlight every morning. This helps re-set your biological clock and will help you fall asleep easier in the evenings.

Quality sleep and proper nutrition are the foundation for looking, feeling and being your best. The combination of the two gives you the fuel you need to balance everything else in your life, and is the key to going forward to claim your own What's Next.

CHAPTER 6: What I've Learned About Healthy Aging

Of all the self-fulfilling prophecies in our culture, the assumption that aging means decline and poor health is probably the deadliest.

— Marilyn Ferguson, *The Aquarian Conspiracy*

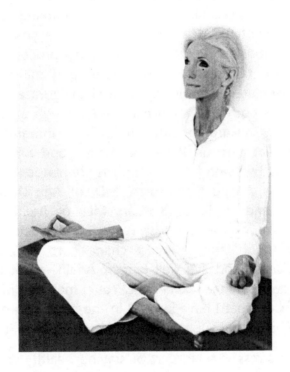

I don't think we can talk about creating What's Next without addressing the all-important subject of our health. After all, we are starting to, or are already facing, health issues we didn't worry about when we were younger. The years of *using* our bodies catch up to us eventually, don't they? Luckily for us, there is more information than ever available that gives us choices when it comes to our health and wellness.

While aging is inevitable, the development of age-related disease is not. We *can* age gracefully, through making choices and choosing behaviors that promote health. The goal is to reach old age through a flexible, balanced approach that leaves us feeling and looking younger for as long as possible.

These ideas remind me of a quote by Karl von Bonstetten: "To resist old age, one must combine the body, the mind and the heart—and to keep them in parallel vigor, one must exercise, study and love." Some of us baby boomers are doing just that, as evidenced by the second careers we are embarking upon and the dreams we continue to follow. Maintaining a youthful spirit is especially important in slowing the aging process. No matter how well we take care of our bodies and minds, if we are spiritually depleted, we will not age well. Invigorate your spirit by keeping your body and mind balanced through practicing well-being! Today we are so fortunate to have integrative medical doctors available to us. It has been my good fortune to have come across two who have helped me tremendously in the last ten years: Dr Arlene Noodleman, MD, of Age Defy in Silicon Valley, CA, and Dr Bruce Berman, MD, of Jupiter, FL. These doctors utilize and respect both Eastern and Western traditions, and have taught me to make changes to promote health, prevent disease and live well longer. Again—what follows has been my own personal experience. Yours may be different, but I want to share what I have learned in the hope and belief that it may be of value and you may learn something from it.

Combating stress is a big part of staying healthy and is one of the first things to enter our minds when we talk about achieving wellness in our lives. Stress is an imbalance of homeostasis that leaves us in varying degrees of disruption. Stress varies from short term cases like public speaking, rush hour traffic and flying on an airplane to life altering stresses like divorce, death of a loved one and job loss. There are times that stress seems inescapable. Maybe it is at times, but we often put more stress on our minds and bodies than we need to...worrying about things that might not (and usually don't) ever happen. Then there are times when it's justified. Figuring out how we react to different levels of stressful situations is a great first step in reducing our overall stress level. Negative thought patterns often go hand-in-hand with stress, leaving us unhealthy in our bodies, minds, and especially our souls.

The problem of Stress

Our spirits become depleted through lifelong negative thought patterns and loss of vitality in all areas of life; in other words, they succumb to internalized "ageism." It's important to correct these patterns, which can be done by learning about the different methods available that increase energy and reduce stress. One effective way to do this is through a Mindfulness-Based Stress Reduction Program. First developed by Jon Kabat Zinn, and based on the ancient Buddhist Practice of Mindfulness, MBSR helps people take an active role in the management of their health, teaching them to become more aware of their thoughts and feelings, and to change their relationship to those thoughts and feelings. These programs have been used not only for personal meditation, but in over two hundred hospitals in the U.S. and around the world. Mindfulness a remarkably effective way to improve not only your thoughts and emotions, but also your overall physical health.

It's universally understood that stress impacts us physically, mentally and emotionally. Because it works from the inside out, it takes a toll on our outermost physical "envelope," the skin—stress can literally be "written all over our faces!" At Age Defy, they call this the 'Complexion Connection.' Making changes to reduce stress and promote a sense of well-being may also decrease the effect of stress on the skin, improving conditions such as acne, rosacea and even eczema. Plus, you'll just look more relaxed!

"Healthy aging"—and not "anti-aging" is the most appropriate and encouraging way to look at turning back the clock when it comes to keeping our skin looking young and bright. But it's not about masking age! It's about maintaining age-appropriate skin as we get older. The focus should always be on following a plan to achieve healthier skin. A natural by-product of that planis that, as the skin becomes healthier, it also looks better. It becomes radiant, smoother and more evenly toned

As Dr. Noodleman says, Eastern and Western approaches can also address the outward signs of aging. Their causes are, in large part, due to oxidative stress and the subsequent production of destructive "free radicals," which result in the three D's: deflation, deterioration and descent. In the West, cosmetic surgery is commonly used to combat the three D's. However, extreme 'makeovers' may result in an unnatural, expression-less look. Some are so overdone that they actually have an almost 'pickled' appearance. Our youth-obsessed society has lost sight of the essential components of aging gracefully: balance and moderation. Outward appearance is over-emphasized while the most important characteristics of youth—energy, resilience, flexibility, balance and strength—are often overlooked.

Top Ten Wellness Facts:

1.   According to the American Institute of Stress, up to 90% of all health problems are related to stress.

2.   Research confirms that our thoughts and emotions have a dynamic effect on our health and vitality.

3.   Acupuncture, mindfulness-based stress reduction, therapeutic massage and energy-based treatments facilitate healing and complement cosmetic dermatology and rejuvenating medi-spa treatments. All activate the body's natural reparative processes, reduce stress and help to achieve a balanced, healthier life.

4.   Scientific studies have found a strong link between the complexion and emotions - activities designed to improve our emotional state have the added benefit of improving the quality of the skin, which in turn decreases stress, further improving our emotional state!

5. The immune system and the body's ability to heal quickly are directly affected by stress and one's overall mind-body health.

6. Consider adopting an anti-inflammatory diet, such as the traditional Japanese or Mediterranean, to promote health and decrease the chances of developing age-related diseases.

7. While baby boomers have aged in years, most haven't aged in spirit. Many are not retiring just to spend their days idly at home. Instead, they're living active lifestyles, traveling, even embarking upon second careers. For them, retirement represents an opportunity to live out their dreams.

9. The goal is to prevent, modify or even reverse the changes that time brings. The best approach is not a denial of the aging process, but rather a choice to delay the onset of age-related decline and disease for as long as possible.

10. Beauty and wellness go hand-in-hand. Your skincare regimen, fitness level and lifestyle choices all affect how you look and feel.

Now for a word from Dr. Bruce Berman, MD. Recently I sat down with Dr. Berman in his office in Jupiter, FL. Dr. Berman is an MD who specializes in holistic and integrative medicine. Following is his own medical opinion, and you should always consult with your own doctor before starting on any new regimen.

> *"Of all the self-fulfilling prophecies in our culture, the assumption that aging means decline and poor health is probably the deadliest."*
>
> - Marilyn Ferguson, *The Aquarian Conspiracy*, 1980

V: What are some of the newest findings that we should know about regarding healthy aging?

Dr. B: The foundation for anti-aging is hormonal balance between the thyroid, adrenal and sex hormones. 95% - 97% of doctors in the U.S. don't know how to diagnose or treat thyroid deficiency. The most accurate way to test for low thyroid is to taking your temperature before rising daily for 10-14 days. A majority of temperatures below 97.4 indicates that you have low thyroid, no matter what blood tests may say. If it turns out that your thyroid is low, the most effective treatment is a specially compounded drug prescribed by your physician based on your test results.

V: What are the most important hormones we should be taking?

Dr B: Estrogen to help protect against Alzheimer's. It also helps your skin, resulting in fewer wrinkles by plumping up subcutaneous fats. Progesterone, the "feel good hormone," balances estrogen and is protective against breast and uterine cancer. In addition, not enough of it causes PMS symptoms.

Women need testosterone too—but they need it differently from men.

Andropause—male menopause—is epidemic in this country. Just replacing testosterone may not be enough. Some patients may need to be on several hormones. Men should be tested to determine deficiencies. Synthetic progesterone produces the opposite effect of bio-identical hormones.

V: How do you recommend that women take their hormones?

Dr. B: I recommend custom compounded bio-identical hormones in troche form, based on individualized blood tests. (A troche is dissolved in the mouth between the gum and the cheek, where it is absorbed into the blood stream).

To find a good holistic/integrative medical doctor, go to www.acam.org - a holistic physicians finder site.

*****

The incomparable George Burns who lived to see his 100th birthday, said, "We can't help getting older, but we can help getting old."

We don't have to look at advancing birthdays with a sense of dread. We can and should continue to look for new opportunities to challenge ourselves, stretch our minds, and look around the corner to see what's next.

Aging gracefully means so many things—not the least of which is loving yourself by taking care of yourself. Looking and feeling your very best takes some effort and discipline, but the rewards are well worth it. A healthy diet, proper exercise, and sleep are all key ingredients. So is a good skin regimen to keep that beautiful glow in your cheeks and the wrinkles at bay.

In short, aging gracefully means being your most vibrant, natural, healthy, well cared for self.

I don't want to end it there, however.... Because if we are to age with joy and vitality, we certainly need to have our fill of all of life's pleasures.... A wonderful meal with friends that includes a bottle of wine and an outrageously decadent dessert, unforgettable evenings where we have lingered on much too late and totally abandoned the seven hours of sleep idea, and days where we skip the gym and go wherever the spirit takes us. Life is meant to be relished and enjoyed to the fullest, creating magnificently happy memories along the way. It means, too, giving of ourselves and sharing the best of what we are with others.

As we go through life, if we can learn to navigate the peaks and valleys with a positive attitude, not allowing negative thoughts and undue stress to get the better of us, we will have gone a long way towards aging with grace.

In conclusion, aging gracefully means arriving at the summit, full of joy and laughter, with love in our hearts, full of gratitude for all of life's gifts, and rich with the wisdom we have acquired along the way. It means having a wealth of happy memories to draw upon and looking forward with eager anticipation to more to come. In other words...To creating What's Next.

CHAPTER 7: The Art of Keeping Sexuality Alive

Happiness comes from the capacity to feel deeply, to enjoy simply, to think freely, to risk life, to be needed.

— Storm Jameson

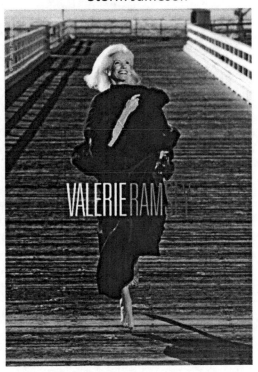

$\mathcal{A}$s I sit here at my desk thinking about the role that sexuality and sensuality play in our lives, my thoughts drift over to the deliciously erotic poems of my dear friend, Minx Boren. Minx has a way of getting to the heart of the deepest connection between two people that is unlike any other. She reads our minds. She knows our deepest feelings. And she expresses them so beautifully. So bear with me. I can't resist.... This would be the perfect time to introduce you to one of Minx's poems. It comes from her book, *Ripe,* which is succulently illustrated by Patti Burris. All of Patti's drawings are depictions of ripe, delicious pears. Enjoy....

do you ever feel

soft

and juicy

like a luscious fruit

warmed

and ripened

to perfection

succulent

basking

in your fullness

wanting

to be savored

imagine

how tantalizing and

delicious

to celebrate this

blossoming

allowing your juiciness

to overflow and

anoint your every word

and gesture

to arouse your creative force

to sweeten each

experience

and enliven

each connection

Don't you love it? Imagine a whole book full of such erotic deliciousness. She is a gift to all of us.

The following is from *Gracefully*—familiar words worth repeating for those of you who have read the book; thoughtful words for the new reader.

At the end of the chapter, you will see a recent interview I had with Lou Paget, ASSECT (www.loupaget.com). There are few who know more about sexuality than she does, or who are better at demystifying it. Meanwhile, from the pages of *Gracefully*.....

If ever there was a meeting ground for body, mind and soul, the connection between two people who are in love with each other certainly is it. So much of sexuality resides in our minds. And when we love someone, it is not their physical being that we fall in love with (although that may well be part of the initial attraction), but it is the essence of their soul that we love. When our deepest feelings and emotions enter the equation, then our spirits soar and our hearts take flight.

Sensuality enriches our souls as much as it enriches our bodies and minds. It is grand in its breadth and scope. The five senses of sexuality (especially when combined): hearing, touching, seeing, feeling and tasting, wrap us up into an intimacy that reaches a dimension outside ourselves. We draw life in as we are nourished by a lover and give love in return.

When these senses are engaged in the myriad of ways that are open to us, when the inhibitions and fears we had when we were younger have given way to relaxation and understanding, that is when our physical relationships can take on a whole new meaning. I think we are so fortunate to be living in a time when sex is no longer considered taboo for women, and seasoned ones at that. Historically, it was something to be swept under the carpet and denied. Now, as a new awareness and a healthy outlook carry us into later years, our sexuality is recognized as being a key element to who we are. It is something we celebrate as being a rich and fulfilling part of the whole life experience. Not only has sexuality been proven to be good for our health, but it enriches our lives in so many other ways. It keeps the sparkle in our eyes, the bounce in our step, and the radiance in our smile. Sexual expression wears many faces. That's one of the things that keeps it lively and interesting. Love has many moods. One encounter may be sweet and tender, another comforting. One may be urgent and impatient, while still another may take on a sense of daring and adventure.

With a smile and a willingness to take a risk, try making love in a brand way in a brand new place. It's hard to get bored if routine doesn't have the chance to set in. As women, it's sometimes easy to fall into a pattern of allowing our lover to be the aggressor, but men love it when we take them by surprise and switch roles on them. They want and need to know that we have needs, too. It's a wonderful reminder for them that there are times when our desires well up just as strongly as theirs do. Men are thrilled and flattered at this idea, and when we open up to them and tell them how we're feeling, it makes the bond that much stronger. Mutual appreciation, caring and loving acts, benefit both partners. Don't make love just for him—fulfill your own desires and needs. The idea is to keep the relationship fresh by being open to all of the different ways in which we can express our sexuality. Communicating sexually in a healthy and established relationship keeps the doors of communication open in other areas as well.

Sexuality energizes us. It makes us radiate with joy just to be alive. As we saw in the chapter on exercise, it's important to stimulate your body to keep it in the best shape possible. The same holds true for your sexuality.

Exploring the five senses of seeing, hearing, tasting, touching, and smelling is a great way to keep your sexuality young and vital. Here are a few ways to get started:

The Importance of Touch

Any or all of the five senses are always there for us, even if the physical act of making love isn't as easy as it once was! Touch is particularly important in times such as this. A tender caress or a relaxing massage can do wonders for both of you. Touch nourishes and heals as much as it comforts and reassures. The importance of the art, yes art, of touching, cannot be emphasized enough.

Indulge your sense of touch. Treat yourself and your partner to a massage—or better yet, indulge in a couple's massage! Buy some nice satiny sheets or a soft wool blanket and enjoy the way it feels against your skin. Indulge in buying some scented lotions or oils, and see the way they feel on your skin, or enjoy the sensation of rubbing them on your partner's body. Take a cool bath on a hot day together, and enjoy the simple way the water feels on your bodies.

Hold hands in the movie theater, touch your partner's shoulder when expressing gratitude or appreciation, and everyone's favorite—run fingers through their hair, or in some cases massage a bald scalp! Put your hand in his pocket while waiting in line. These gestures shouldn't be wasted on the young!

Intimate gestures. Reminding touches. Soft touches. Those are the moments of touch.

The Importance of Taste

Sharing a meal with a cherished partner or friend is another way our senses are engaged and intimacy is fostered. Inhaling the delicious aromas, sipping a glass of wine, and spending time with friends and loved ones is truly one of life's greatest pleasures. The simple act of being together, of opening up to each other in meaningful conversation and hearty laughter has a warming and relaxing affect on us. Appreciating the humor in life as we share our experiences encourages intimacy. It is in the act of sharing, of being together and giving each other our undivided attention, that we open the door to our inner selves and invite intimacy in. When we share our thoughts and make ourselves available to others, we are allowing and encouraging them to do the same. This is how we connect, and I believe that connection is the key element to creating a rich and happy life.

Take the time to have dinner together—linger over a long meal and just talk about your day together; make it a rule not to talk about your jobs or your families for a few hours and just try to focus on one another; make a meal that has particular importance to you—perhaps it's something you used to cook together when you were once a poor, newly married couple, or a meal that will remind you of a nice vacation you once had; or go out to dinner at a special restaurant as you did on one of your first dates, etc. Feed each other dessert—be a bit playful. And if some whipped cream or some chocolate sauce follows you into the bedroom, then so be it!

Food is not only about taste, but also about other senses such as smell and even touch. Different foods have different textures that we can react to positively, neutrally or negatively and the combination of texture and taste makes a big difference. Similarly, the taste of your partner's lips is one of the most intimate tastes in the world. You can identify them blindfolded not only because of their taste, but their feel—how they feel on your own lips, neck and shoulders. When we increase our understanding of how taste in other areas of life can influence our senses, sensuality reaches new levels. Have fun and experiment!

The Sounds of Love

Few things spark our imagination the way music does. It has the power to speak to our soul, to light up our hearts, to fuel our energy, to bring back a flood of memories and to open the gates

67

to creating new ones. It can charge us up as we race out into a brand new day, and at the end of the day it can relax us. Music transports us into a mood of intimacy as it feeds and awakens our senses. It has the power to release an immensely strong emotional response, making us want to dance or cry, sing along in joy or tear up at a memory so vivid that it's as if it happened yesterday. Nothing sets a mood the way music does. Nothing communicates a mood the way music does. Nothing speaks of romance the way music does.

The same can be said for the written word, especially when it is spoken aloud, whether it is great literature, a love letter, or a whispered fantasy! Few things are more romantic or touch the heart as deeply as a poem written by a lover to his beloved, the more personal and original, the better. It needn't be Emily Dickinson or Robert Browning. The expression of feelings is what matters, the caring and thought that went into the act of writing it. The way it says, "I love you;" or, sometimes, "I want you." Any woman will tell you that a poem or a love letter, even those three little words scrawled on a cocktail napkin, can be profoundly touching. She will also tell you that it is this type of foreplay that leads to the greatest and most satisfying sexual encounters of all.

Play some of your favorite old songs, or some music that reminds you of a particular time in your life. Go to a concert together or sing a song that the two of you used to love.

It's not only music that can make us relax and put us in a romantic mood. Recite a poem to your partner, one that conveys your true inner self. Tell your man how attractive you find him, how he is still handsome to you after all of these years; tell him specifically what parts of him—his strong arms, his head of hair, his calloused hands—you find most attractive. Be a bit daring—share a sexual fantasy with him, or tell him how you've been thinking about him all day and what you imagined the two of you doing together as soon as he got home, etc.

No matter where we live, when we go on vacation there are always new sounds, and sometimes it's the lack of sound that's different. A beach vacation allows the rhythm of waves hypnotically crashing on the shore, whereas a vacation in the city allows the hustle and bustle of action and excitement emanating from the streets. These different sounds alone remind us that we are in a new environment and give us an opportunity to explore our reactions to these sounds. Both coming in from a day on the beach or returning from a Broadway show leave new sounds in your conscious and subconscious. The hypnotic waves can relax and set the scene for a romantic evening just as easily as the symphony of the city. It's all what you make of them while in their setting.

Beauty is in the Eye of The Beholder

The power of sight when it comes to sensuality and sexuality is quite powerful. For some, the gesture of looking into one another's eyes or simply noticing the allure of a five o'clock shadow is enough to arouse. Others are visually inspired by the curve in a muscle or the way hair falls across the face. We all have our favorites!

What we take in visually on any given day can have such an impact on our moods and emotions that by the time we get home sensory overload has taken over. Reduce the overload by focusing on a simple yet favorite visual. Maybe it's a photograph or painting you love. Allow yourself a moment to just sit and look at it. Think about the calming emotions the image evokes and allow the positive energy to replace the mayhem of the day. Meditation often uses an object as a visual reference to focus on...such as a flickering candle. It's calming and the bunched up sensory overload can melt away in minutes, changing your mood and refocusing your needs.

Indulge your sense of sight by going to a movie together, or driving up to the top of a mountain to enjoy the view and sit silently together or alone, soaking up all the natural beauty around you. Perhaps go to the local video store and rent a romantic or explicitly sexual movie—enjoy watching it together, and see where it might take you! Buy some sexy clothes that will make you look and feel sexy—dim the lights a little bit, and let your partner get in the mood by letting him watch you.

It All Comes Down to Chemistry

The power of chemistry between two people can't be overemphasized. Without it, everything else falls by the wayside. It's an inexplicable magic that draws the two of you together with a power and a force that can't be defined or ignored. It is the electricity that crackles through to the core of our being at the sound of a lover's voice, at the laughter that crinkles his eyes. It is the fire in a touch, the warmth in an embrace. It is that magical force that makes making love the wondrous and beautiful thing that it is. It may seem to slip away with the passage of time, but in a strong and loving relationship, it never disappears entirely. It simply lies dormant, ready to spring to life again when given proper attention.

Appreciating your partner involves saying I love you, showing your feelings in a thousand little ways, and never taking each other for granted. Women, especially, never tire of hearing the words, "I love you." Maybe it's a Mars and Venus thing, but women desire and need validation. Men, too, thrive on genuine validation and knowing they're appreciated. It's only human to want to know that we are needed, appreciated and loved. I never hang up the phone with a family member or close friend without saying, "I love you." To me, it's so important to always let them know how valued they are and how much I treasure having them in my life.

Enthusiasm is Everything

Let's face it—as we approach middle age and beyond, our bodies no longer look the way they did when we were in our twenties. We may have added a few pounds and changed in all sorts of ways we never thought we would when we were younger, and that can take its toll on our confidence in the bedroom. Whereas we never gave making love with the lights on a moment's thought before, the very thought may now fill us with dread and embarrassment. I was recently asked the question, "What do you say to a woman who is fearful of having her lover or partner see her naked because she's self-conscious about a "pooch" or unwanted pounds in places where she never used to have them?" My answer is this: "If you are filled with enthusiasm about being together—if you open your arms wide and greet him with a big smile and a warm embrace, letting him know that there is no one else in the whole world that you would rather be with, and that you can't wait to have him come to bed with you," then believe me, he won't care. He won't even notice! And besides— chances are his body has seen a few changes over the years as well. Remember—it's not about how we look; it's about how we make our partners feel, and if we make them feel wonderful about themselves, then believe me, nothing else matters.

Everything we have written about throughout this book is an important component to sexuality. If you are fit and strong, you feel sexier. If you have self-confidence, you feel sexier. If you feel good about your body, faults and all, and are tuned into your own sensuality, you definitely feel sexier. If you are open, loving and have a good sense of humor, that is sexy. Power is sexy. Success is sexy. Glamour is sexy. So are honesty, vulnerability, tenderness, sweetness, and enthusiasm. Nothing is sexier or more irresistible than a lover who truly wants and desires you and whom you truly want and desire in return. Find what works between the two of you, and continuously explore these and other ways to keep your love and love life alive.

Sexuality is not just about ourselves. What it really is about is the way in which we open ourselves to another and connect on the deepest level. It's when we move outside ourselves and into the realm of a lover that our most meaningful connections take place. It's when we care more about someone else than we do ourselves. And it's when we no longer concern ourselves so much with the outcome as we do with the journey. If fireworks go off at the end of the road, beautiful, but if not, then that's all right too. The act of intimacy is so important: the touching, the caring, the tenderness, the sense of adventure, the trust you have in one another, looking into each other's eyes and realizing yet again how very lucky you are to have this person in your life and to be giving yourself in this way. Surrender yourself and strive to not be afraid to try something new and then, when you do, if it turns out to be awkward or is just plain doesn't work out, laugh about it. Life is often funny, and so is human sexuality! Again, it's about love and laughter, of allowing humor and happiness to bubble up and create your joy.

A few years ago when *Gracefully* first came out, I was invited to go up to Toronto to be a presenter at the annual CARP conference, "A New Vision of Aging," put on by The Canadian Association of Retired Persons. They had invited Thought Leaders from a variety of fields, and I met so many interesting people! Most were Canadians, but there were a few of us from the U.S., two of whom I have been in touch with ever since. One was Dr. Michael Breus, PhD, an internationally recognized sleep specialist who speaks all over the world and has appeared on numerous television shows in the U.S.—Dr. Oz, Oprah, The Doctors, Katie, and many others. See www.thesleepdoctor.com. (Chapter 5, Advice from the Sleep Doctor). The other was Lou Paget, also internationally known, a popular speaker and best-selling author of five books on sexuality (see www.loupaget.com). Lou is an AASECT Certified Sex Educator. She is someone whom sex therapists learn from.

To quote from her website, "Lou is a researcher whose quest for accurate, practical information for herself has created a highly successful international seminar and product company with a focus on lifestyle and cultural trends that impact our sexuality, health, and relationships." I remember when the CARP sponsor, Moses Xaimer of Zoomer Media, introduced her, he said, "Everything Lou says, she can say with her pearls on." Lou is so knowledgeable and articulate, while at the same time very warm and funny, that one feels comfortable discussing the most intimate subjects with her.

Taking again from her website, because it states her mission so perfectly, "With her trademark calm and fearless intelligence, Paget delivers the core essence of information about intimacy. As an international bestselling author of five books, translated into twenty-six languages, and represented in over sixty countries with over three million copies sold, it is clear that global audiences are hungry for Paget's expertise. When it comes to intimacy and sexuality, Paget says, 'Common sense isn't all that commonly practiced, but we all want it.'"

When I speak, particularly to men and women over 50, I am often asked questions that need an informed answer, and that is when I will turn to Lou. I recently had such a discussion with her, and I would like to share what we talked about because I think our conversation is reflective of what so many would like to ask her if they had her sitting in their living rooms. I will go down the list of the topics we discussed:

V—You have been speaking and writing about sexuality since the '90's. What changes have you seen over the last twenty years, particularly now that so many women have entered the workforce? How has their success and confidence impacted their sex lives?

L—Actually we know women have been in the workforce long before the 90's; however, what I have seen change over the last twenty years is more women delaying marriage, choosing relationship styles that suit them; e.g., living together, blending families without marriage. Yet most important is the career minded single woman, and married woman who is making more money in the household, and Honey, when you control the wallet, you control a lot; translation: you have a voice and a confidence. AND having a voice carries from the boardroom to the bedroom. Marketers of sex toys, marital aids, which ever term you prefer, know this and know women are choosing what they like and want sexually, partnered or not. So once partnered, these women bring their confidence and awareness of their sexual self and script into their relationship.

V—What you say is so true, Lou. I went from being a stay-at-home wife and mother throughout the '60's, '70's and '80's, to entering the corporate world in '93. I loved those years at home and wouldn't have traded them for anything, but it wasn't until I got out in the world and proved myself outside of the framework of domesticity, that I truly came into my own. I gained a self-confidence that I had never had before.

V—What else has changed over the years? I have a lot of people tell me that their sexual drive has greatly diminished. Why do you suppose that is?

L—Huge question and one that doesn't have a simple answer. The answers to this question create a tapestry, one with many threads, colors and hues. I'll quickly run through what I ask people so they can do a personal review: 1) Are you bored/uninterested/irritated by your partner? If so, you need to address those issues before you can truly show up intimately with a partner. 2) How much stress is in your life? E.g., for men the stress hormone cortisol works in direct opposition to testosterone. Are you a squeezed woman who works, is dealing with kids at home and aging parents? 3) Medications you're taking...don't expect your physician to know how these drugs impact your sexual health and libido. Remember that generally speaking, they are trained by pharma representatives. Are you taking any medications for anxiety, depression? Blood pressure meds? Lipitor? Did you take oral birth control? FYI—walking outside for 30 minutes has been shown to be as beneficial, if not more so, than anti-depressive meds.

Asexuality - There are some people who love another deeply and are attracted to a person yet have no sexual interest. They had a sexual interest and then zip.

Hormonal changes - For some women when the estrogen drops during menopause and perimenopause, it is as though their sex drive took a holiday.

V—I often hear from women who have been in a relationship for a long time that their partner no longer has interest in them. It can work the other way around too—the woman may lose any feeling of attraction she once had for her man. Can this be reversed?

L –Of course—but with some work and awareness. Here's some great news from the work of Dr. Rosemary Basson. For many women their sex drive doesn't kick in UNTIL they are being sexually engaged. Translation: their libido is jump-started by sexual action, unlike male libido that is the drive. So for women when their brain is engaged, their body follows suit. Let's also be clear in our understanding that desire and sexual interest can encompass a broad range of activities, not simply intercourse. The important thing is to always remember that you, and only you, can know what you like, and only you can give your partner attention. If you aren't paying attention to your relationship, someone or something else will because human beings need attention.

V—Let's take a look at the subject of hormones.

L—A huge topic!!! Before I start I ask people to be their own shrewd consumer. Find a health care provider that matches your philosophy about this and keep on educating yourself about products. One of the saddest things in my mind was the Women's Health Initiative that started with such promise and then due to poor study setups and the manner in which the ensuing 'results' were interpreted, many women mistakenly ran from hormone replacement therapy—the very therapy that was helping them thorough the rocky parts of perimenopause and menopause. A fun easy reading book is by Ellen Dolgen, who is that friend who researched the hormone options when she was slammed into menopause and lost her sex drive. She waded through the morass of information on female hormone replacement and delivers it in her book *Shimersky*.

V—In the area of sensuality and sexuality, how do you keep this alive in a relationship?

L—Attention, attention, attention. Your attention is your most seductive gift, and given how many encounters we have with others, some of whom we find attractive because they are 'new,' it's up to each of us, individually and together, to nurture our relationship. Truly, I have seen that respect is the number one behavior that is an indicator of a relationship's stability or how a person will be in a relationship. Love is great, yet respect is the big one. I love this comment: A man married many decades was asked by an interviewer how he kept his relationship strong? He answered, "That's simple. Whenever I thought the grass was greener on the other side, I started watering my grass." Love it!!!

V—Sometimes I feel uncomfortable bringing up the subject of sexuality in front of an audience for fear that there may be people there who are without partners. I don't want to offend them or make them feel that they are missing out. How do you recommend that I handle this?

L—Don't shy away from this subject. We are all born of sexuality. It defines almost everything we do, so even if they don't have a partner now, address and deliver information inclusively, as they are likely to have one in the future. Being single by event or choice is a cycle for many people throughout their lives. What doesn't change is people seeking out people who make them feel good. So partnered or not, sometimes the best sex people have is solo sex as they know exactly what is going to work. Then should they choose, they can share that with a partner. Relationships, sexuality and sensuality, are all about choice. Choose often, choose well and choose wisely.

I asked Lou which of her five books best addressed the questions we had just discussed, and she recommended *The Great Lover Playbook*. Lou gave me this book as a gift a few years ago, and I agree—it is both excellent and informative. I highly recommend it too.

To learn more about Lou, please see www.loupaget.com

CHAPTER 8: Beautiful on the Outside

A Girl Should Be Two Things: Classy And Fabulous.

— Coco Chanel

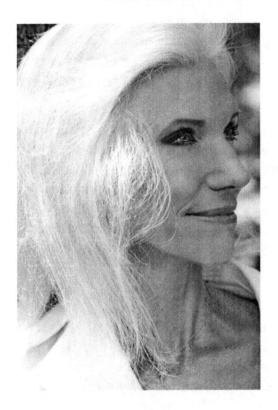

Whenever I speak, I like to open the floor to a Q&A session afterwards. When this happens, I am invariably asked about two things: my beauty routine and my hair! I have a routine with preferred products for hair and skin that is fairly simple and works consistently for me now; however, it has changed over the years as I've aged. One of the most important things to realize when it comes to beauty is that it's not about the money you spend as much as it is about finding the products that work best for your skin and hair types and then combining them to achieve the best results for you. It is very important to understand that skin and hair change as we age, so watch for products that may no longer work as well as they once did and be willing to make changes.

Not only is it about what products you choose, and the amount, but the key is how you <u>apply</u> a product. For example, a twenty-year-old applies make-up with a much different goal than a sixty-year-old. In our youth we apply make-up to be noticed and to enhance what nature has already provided -almost as an art form.

But, as we grow older, we use make-up to enhance features, play down noticeable defects such as under eye circles or uneven coloring, and to maintain a healthy and radiant appearance. A younger woman's advantages are her plump pink lips, rosy cheeks, bright eyes, smooth skin, and glossy hair; whereas, when we age, the natural fading of these characteristics needs to be overcome by the application of products that bring that healthy look back.

Skin Care

Wouldn't it be nice to have the skin of a twenty year old again! Sadly, that's not going to happen any time soon. The fact is, aging skin is unavoidable, but there are things you can do to keep your skin—and the rest of your face—looking young and healthy.

But first, some facts on why skin ages the way it does, from my dear friend, Dr. Alberto Pena, MD.

How Does Skin Change With Age?

As you approach your 30s, your body's production of collagen and elastin (two substances that give the skin firmness and elasticity) begins to slow down. The collagen and elastin also begin to loosen and unravel which results in skin that is looser and less supple.

At the same time, fat cells beneath the skin may begin to disappear. With the loss of this supportive fat, collagen, and elastin, plus the pull of gravity, the skin begins to sag and form wrinkles. It also loses the ability to moisturize itself and retain moisture, leading to dryness, possibly with itchy, irritated patches.

With age also comes the appearance of those familiar lines and wrinkles that we associate with older skin; frown lines (those between the eyebrows) and crow's feet (lines that radiate from the corners of the eyes) begin to appear as a result of permanent small muscle contractions.

Your Habits, Your Skin

In addition to the natural processes that occur in our bodies and skin as we age, other long-term habits can cause damage to our skin. You will want to reduce your exposure to sun, the most damaging external factor that affects the condition and health of our skin and is the primary cause of premature aging (called photoaging) and skin cancers (including melanoma, basal cell carcinoma, and squamous cell carcinoma). In fact, many of the features we associate with aged skin are actually caused by sun exposure, and not by the natural aging process. Photoaging can cause a number of skin conditions, including:

- Fine wrinkles
- Liver spots (a.k.a. age spots)
- Dilated blood vessels

Smoking cigarettes is also harmful to the skin. Smoking causes the blood vessels in the top layers of the skin to narrow (constrict), which reduces the blood supply, reduces the amount of oxygen available to the skin, and reduces the removal of waste products and dead cells. This process contributes to the reduction in collagen and elastin and prevents Vitamin A from bonding with skin cells to repair skin damage, leading skin to have a grayish or bluish cast and a leathery texture. Smoking also restricts circulation, taking away the rosy blush of young skin. The facial expressions smokers make when smoking may also cause wrinkles around lips (pursing around a cigarette) and around eyes (squinting to keep out smoke).

One of the most important things you can do for your skin is to eat a diet high in antioxidants and omega-3 fatty acids. Salmon, tuna, mackerel, and lake trout are all high in natural omega-3 oils. Leafy green vegetables and brightly colored fruits are great sources of antioxidants: spinach, broccoli, tomatoes, strawberries and blueberries are all excellent choices. The deeper the color, the better it is for you.

Common Signs of Aging Skin

When skin ages and accumulates damage from sun and other habits, a number of skin conditions may result including:

- Lentigines - Also known as "age" or "liver" spots, lentigines are flat, brown spots that usually show up on the face, hands, back and feet. These spots are not dangerous (and are not a sign of liver disease). If, however, you notice a dark, flat area with irregular (not rounded) borders, see a dermatologist to ensure that it is not a melanoma.
- Bruises - Older skin bruises more often than younger skin and takes a much longer time to heal. Bruises that don't heal after a week or so should be seen by a dermatologist.
- Wrinkles - As skin becomes less elastic, it begins sag, particularly around the eyes, mouth, forehead, and cheeks.
- Telangiectasias - Often called "broken capillaries," telangiectases are visible, dilated blood vessels in the face, usually caused by sun damage.
- Actinic keratoses - These are rough, warty, reddish or brownish growths, caused by sun damage and are often a precursor to squamous cell carcinoma (skin cancer).
- Cherry Angiomas- These are red, protruding growths on the body caused by dilated blood vessels. They are

harmless and occur in about 85% of those over middle-aged.

- Seborrheic Keratoses - These are brown or black raised spots, or warty growths on the skin's surface

Keep Your Skin Looking Younger

It's best to start protecting your skin during childhood; however, anyone at any age can begin to take the necessary precautions to help protect the skin, keep it looking young and healthy, and hopefully slow down the affects of aging. Following are some tips on how to achieve younger looking skin.

- Minimize Sun Exposure - Minimizing sun exposure is the most important thing you can do to protect your skin and keep it looking young. Wear sunscreen of at least SPF 15 when outdoors, and protect the face with a brimmed hat. Try to avoid sun exposure from approximately 10:00 AM to 4:00 PM, which is the most hazardous time for UV exposure.
- Protect Skin From Dryness - Aging skin can be dry, flaking and itchy. Use a moisturizer containing petrolatum or lanolin immediately after bathing. Also, use milder soaps and consider bathing less often and using less drying warm water to bathe rather than hot water.
- Drink Plenty of Water - Drinking water throughout the day ensures proper hydration of the body and helps to reduce skin dryness. Doctors and nutritionists recommend drinking at least 6-8 glasses of water every day.
- Eat a Healthy Diet - Eating a healthy, balanced diet will benefit your body as well as your skin. Fruits and vegetables are particularly important for preventing premature skin aging since they contain many antioxidants

- Exercise - Exercise promotes capillary functioning, which can decrease premature aging. It also increases oxygen to the tissues, which keeps skin looking young and healthy.
- Stop Smoking - Quitting smoking at any age reduces further damage to skin.

Product Helpers

Following are some common active ingredients in over-the-counter products that can help keep your skin looking young and healthy:

- Alpha-Hydroxy Acids (AHAs) - These acids produce a mild sloughing (peeling) action, taking off the top layer of skin and exposing the fresher skin underneath. AHAs are usually derived from fruit or from dairy products, and many moisturizers now contain them. They are safe to use on the face. These are sometimes called "lactic acid" if they're derived from dairy products.
- Retinol - Related to Vitamin A, retinol is contained in many skin creams, and may temporarily cause tissues of the face to swell very slightly, reducing the appearance of fine lines and wrinkles.
- Antioxidants - Topical antioxidant vitamins such as Vitamins C and E can help cells repair the damage caused by the sun's ultraviolet radiation and smoking. This can help skin appear smoother and more glowing.
- Ammonium Lactate - The combination of lactic acid mixed with ammonium hydroxide, ammonium lactate is used to clear up dry, scaly patches on the skin.
- Ceramide - This substance is beginning to play a large part in creams intended to make skin look younger. Ceramide helps the skin hang on to its natural moisturizing lipids and helps reduce damage to skin cells.
- Gingko Biloba - This natural herbal concentrate is not scientifically proven but claims to increase circulation, making skin appear more rosy and clear.

- Another substance, tretinoin, is related to Vitamin A and retinol. Tretinoin cream, currently available only by prescription, can be used on the face to treat acne, fine wrinkles, rough skin and mottled pigmentation.

Healthy Skin Regimen

Nurturing healthy skin is actually a relatively simple process. It's as easy as cleansing properly, exfoliating and moisturizing

Step 1: Clean Your Skin

As women, we are forever making new discoveries and getting introduced to new products that have just come on the market (which they seem to do at an increasingly rapid rate). One such major discovery has come to my attention just within the last year, although this product line has been around a few years longer than that. I am referring to the Rodan + Fields Redefine line. For those of you who haven't heard of this, Katie Rodan, MD, and Kathy Fields, MD, are the two Stanford-trained dermatologists who are also behind the wildly successful Proactiv Solution that was first introduced in 1995 for the treatment of acne. Five years ago they developed a new line of products— Redefine Regimen for the Appearance of Lines, Pores and Loss of Firmness– this one to help prevent and correct the visible signs of aging and restore a firmer, smoother, more youthful-looking complexion. This is a simple 4-product line, consisting of the Daily Cleansing Mask, the Pore Minimizing Toner, the Triple Defense Treatment SPF30, and the Overnight Restorative Cream. I have found these products to be extremely effective. I also love the Redefine MACRO Exfoliator. These products really do keep my complexion glowing, even toned, and healthy looking.

Step 2: Toner

Once my face is nice and clean, I like to use a toner to tighten my pores—this also helps get rid of the discoloration that can appear on our skin as we age. I'll use either the Rodan + Fields

Pore Minimizer Toner, or one I like from Clinique. I recommend that you use a very mild form of toner that contains virtually no alcohol (0-10%), water, and a humectant such as glycerine. Humectants help to keep the moisture in the upper layers of the epidermis by preventing it from evaporating. Rosewater is a natural and wonderfully fragrant toner.

Skin tonics are slightly stronger and contain a small quantity of alcohol (up to 20%), water and a humectant ingredient. Orange flower water is an example of a skin tonic. Skin tonics are suitable for use on normal, combination, and oily skin, but tend to be harsher than the more gentle toners. I recommend that you avoid harsh astringent toners. These are the strongest form of toner and contain a high proportion of alcohol (20-60%), antiseptic ingredients, water, and a humectant ingredient. These are commonly recommended for oily skins as they are drying, but note that the removal of oil from the skin can lead to excess oil production as the skin tries to compensate for this and prevent moisture loss. Witch hazel is an example of an astringent. To prevent dehydration, astringent is best applied only to problem areas of skin, such as spots.

Step 3: Moisturize, Moisturize, Moisturize!
With advancing age, skin can lose essential moisture, resulting in age spots, wrinkles and dullness. Many moisturizers on the market are specially designed to give your skin immediate luminosity and minimize the appearance of age spots and wrinkles with light-diffusing properties. Since it is essential to protect your skin from the sun, make sure that your moisturizer has an SPF value of 15 or higher. While most people understand the importance of moisturizing their skin, it's just as important to use the right moisturizer. In the winter, choose a cream rather than a lotion, and look for one that is fragrance free. Also, be sure to apply moisturizers immediately after you shower, while the skin is still damp, as well as before and after you spend time in the cold air.

Step 4: The Eyes Have It

Another essential part of my anti-aging routine is eye-cream. There are many to choose from, and they are a good investment to make—they really can help to tighten the skin around the eyes and reduce the appearance of wrinkles. At night I like to use Rodan + Fields Eye Cream, and for day, one that I like is Olay Regenerist Eye Lifting Serum, but any crème that has a bit of Alpha-hydroxy and retin-A will be fine.

Step5: Finishing Touches

It's important not to overdo makeup as we get older. I like using a light foundation to even out my skin tone, and then black mascara and an eyebrow pencil-- well-shaped eyebrows frame the eyes and can make all the difference in your face. Too often, especially if our face has grown paler with age, and our hair a little (or in my case, a lot!) whiter, the overall effect can be one of looking "washed out." So even just a touch of color to offset the color of your eyes, or to emphasize a nice brow line can really enhance the way you look. Eyebrow specialist Anastasia Soare of Anastasia Beverly Hills has been on Oprah several times and is known for saying, "My goal is to make the eyebrows beautifully symmetrical because even when features are asymmetrical—as they most often are—well-shaped brows will bring a kind of harmony to the face." Her products are available online as well. There are many salons where you can get advice on the proper shaping and care of your brows. Take advantage of them! As we age, the best shape and color for our brows might change since our skin and muscle tone have altered.

I use a soft pink lipstick with a touch of gloss over it. Some authorities disagree and recommend reds or corals to brighten the face. As with all make up, you should aim to look your age, just better. Heavy, sharp or bright red lipstick might be fine when you are in your 20s and 30s, but when you are older, it can look cartoonish.

And then the one product I really couldn't live without—well, two actually: a light brushing of bronzer across my cheeks with a pop

87

of pink on the apples. You wouldn't believe how this one simple step can brighten your face and make your eyes shine!

The Crowning Jewel: The Hair

Even though I covered this in such detail in my first book, I'm going to repeat it here for those of you who haven't read it because it seems that I am always being asked about my hair! I used to highlight my light-brown hair throughout my 20's, 30's, 40's and 50's until it started turning increasingly white across the top. Finally, in my early 60's, I just let the white take over and haven't looked back. I am often stopped in the street by women who want to know who colors my hair. Nature, I tell them. If I weren't blessed with such a great color, I would certainly add something to correct and improve it. Don't be afraid of letting your hair go gray or white as long as the color enlivens your face. Your hairdresser can advise you as to which products are good for white or gray hair. If you choose to color it, follow the same tips as you would with make-up by using a clear and subtle color that works with your skin and hair texture. Deep black, bright red or brassy blonde is best left to those in their 20s or 30s. Strive for mellow browns, auburns and blonde.

I've allowed my hair to remain long over the years. It's shoulder length because it works well for me, but everyone should wear a style that is most flattering to their face, height and build—never what you think you should wear because you're a certain age. A good cut is critical so that it falls into place even after being out on a windy day. Combined with suitable color and products to keep your hair manageable and healthy, you will always look your best.

Special Advice for Thinning Hair

Here are some questions and answers that women have asked me regarding their thinning hair:

Q. What hair length best hides thinning hair?

A. Shorter cuts — above the shoulder — work best to camouflage thinning hair. The best hair length for thinning hair also depends on the texture and the style of the hair. Hair that's curly could be cut into layers. Wavy hair could be cut mid-length or long, whereas straight hair could be cut in layers, graduated or blunt, to give volume.

Q. Are some colors better than others at hiding thinning hair?

A. Lighter shades that are closer to the skin tone work best to camouflage thinning hair. Darker shades tend to show a greater contrast, thereby exaggerating the condition.

Q. Does coloring or highlighting hair contribute to further thinning?

A. Since experts tell us that hair thinning is caused by a genetic condition called androgenetic alopecia, and since coloring and highlighting are external applications to the hair shaft, these processes do not contribute to further thinning. If your hair thinning is especially bad, you may wish to consult with your health care provider before coloring your hair.

Q. I'm afraid to go into a salon for a haircut because I am embarrassed that my hair is thinning. What should I do?

A. Don't be worried at all. Most stylists are familiar with all kinds of hair textures and conditions and know the best cuts, colors, and treatment options to help you manage your fine or thinning hair. Remember that your stylist is a professional and is there to help you and offer you advice on how to look your best.

Q. It doesn't seem to matter if I part my hair to the left or to the right — it still shows my thinning scalp. What should I do?

A. Try cutting your hair short and wearing a "messy" style, or try a zigzag part. If the hair is straight, layer the top or layer throughout, and then set with curls to camouflage the thinning. You can also try combing your hair back, with no part.

Q. Does exposure to the sun make hair thinning worse?

A. No, the sun will not make hair thinning worse, but it is a good idea to protect your scalp from the sun with a hat or sunscreen.

Q. Are there special shampoos or conditioners I should use if my hair is thinning?

A. There are many volumizing shampoos and conditioners on the market that will help to plump up fine hair, and some of these may also help the appearance of thinning hair. Also, products containing panthenol and herbs such as jasmine, angelica, and willow will keep your hair looking healthy and full. You should use a shampoo that cleanses your scalp well and a conditioner that is light and won't weigh down hair. Rogaine® is a line of products that addresses the needs of women with fine, thin, and thinning hair.

Q. Does blow-drying my hair contribute to its thinning?

A. No, but sometimes the hair is delicate and fine, so use low heat and less tension. Extreme heat and hard pulling will damage the hair and cause breakage.

Q. I want to use Women's Rogaine to treat my thinning hair. How do I incorporate it into my styling regimen?

A. You can continue to style and care for your hair the same way you always have. Women's Rogaine needs to remain on your scalp for about four hours, so if you're going to wash your hair, wash it and towel-dry it before applying Women's Rogaine to your scalp. Wait for Women's Rogaine to dry, and then just style your hair as you normally would.

Q. How does Women's Rogaine affect my hairstyle? Does it make my hair greasy?

A. Women's Rogaine has the consistency of water and is applied only to the scalp. Applying it to the scalp, twice daily as directed, should not affect your hairstyle or make your hair greasy.

*****

Ladies—when all is said and done—remember this:

Happy girls are pretty girls. Smile, laugh, spread joy, and be happy!

CHAPTER 9: The Importance Of Dressing Well

Simplicity is the keynote of all true elegance.

— Coco Chanel

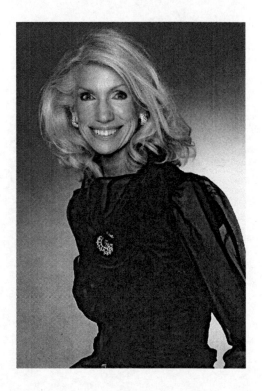

Dressing Well

The way we dress is a strong reflection of who we are. Whether it's an interview, a cocktail party, an opening, or even dropping the kids off at school, when you're dressed properly, you feel good about yourself. You feel confident and you can concentrate on others. When we feel good about ourselves, everything else becomes easier. We are, indeed, expressing our best selves.

What exactly do I mean by "dressing well?" It's simply this—I mean dressing appropriately for your age and lifestyle, looking for quality when you go shopping, and for the most part, sticking to classics. Let's elaborate:

Dressing Appropriately

We've all seen older women who think they look younger if they wear a mini skirt or their teenager's jeans and t-shirt. This look, in my opinion, tops the list of fashion Don'ts. The message it conveys is the exact opposite of the way you want to be perceived. Dress for your body type, age, lifestyle, and the occasion. There are so many excellent choices out there. Dressing for your age doesn't mean "dowdy." It means classic, simple, and beautiful. "Classic" is an individual thing. For the busy career woman, it's usually a well-cut suit, jacket and skirt or dress—in a solid color. For the "soccer mom" it could be well-cut jeans or pants with a great looking blazer or sweater, and loafers. It would NOT be sweat pants or a sweatshirt! When I was working at Pebble Beach, classic for me usually translated into khaki pants with a navy or tweed blazer. After all, it was a golf resort. Shopping for this kind of classic look was simple and fun. I would find khakis that fit perfectly, (usually requiring the assistance of a tailor at my local cleaners to achieve this,) and then add blazers and jackets as I came across them. They did not need to be expensive, but they did need to be of good quality and again, fit perfectly. (I was often able to pick up great looking pieces when my favorite department or specialty stores had their sales). I still wear jackets that I've had in my closet for fifteen years or more, and they always look great because they are timeless and classic.

One more point worth making here has to do with "investment dressing." This is when you buy a "little black dress," or a suit, coat or jacket that will be your "go to" piece. These garments are always of the best quality you can afford, and they have a classic look that never goes out of style. Consider the way the French women dress—they invest in pieces that are of such good style and quality that they last for years and always look right. They may not buy often, but they buy wisely.

Look the Part

Naturally, as we age, the lights in the department store dressing rooms are less forgiving than they were in our youth. Finding clothes that fit properly can make a world of difference. Experiment when you're shopping and find clothes that make you feel and look your best. There are many segments on daytime television, as well as entire television shows, books, and magazines that dedicate their time to showing us how to dress for different body types and how to improve and enhance our images. Clothes can make a tremendous difference in enhancing our self-confidence. When we find clothes that fit properly and are flattering, our whole persona changes and we project our best and most confident selves. Dressing right for an occasion allows us to feel prepared rather than insecure, and we can focus on the occasion with confidence. So many of the old rules have changed and attire expectations tend to be more relaxed than they once were, but keep in mind that relaxed doesn't mean lax.

Accenting Accessories

Accessories are what make any outfit. They complete a look and are one way of expressing our individuality. The possibilities in jewelry choices are limitless. Just recently I discovered the unique designs of Stephanie Kantis. Her beautiful pieces are reflective of her passion for history and travel. Primarily made of bronze dipped in 24k gold, she incorporates semi-precious stones, pearls, quartz and crystal into her pieces. Everything she does has an architectural element to it, resulting in a classic, yet modern, esthetic. I have several of her stunning neckpieces, cuffs, bangles, and unique rings—each and every one a statement piece.

I also love big, handsome, one-of-a-kind pieces of jewelry that are fun and round out jewelry selections. There are many designers around the country who make very handsome costume jewelry, and they're usually available in high-end department stores and boutiques or even trunk shows. These pieces can be signature and statement pieces just as well anything else. Have fun with it. Mix what you like and be open to style possibilities. When I lived in the northeast, I tended to wear gold (costume or real) and pearls, but now that I'm down in south Florida where everything is reflective of the bright sunshine and tropical flowers and greenery, I love fabulous chunky neck pieces that are made of crystal, quartz, and semi-precious stones and that work well with the pinks, greens, blues, whites and yellows that now dominate my wardrobe.

Shoes

Well, don't we all love shoes? And don't we all agree that a shoe can make or break an outfit? And don't we also know that the shoes you wear can speak volumes about who you are? Of course we do! I have worn everything from flip flops to Manolos, and I can see why a woman would be positively thrilled to have a pair of high end designer shoes in her closet. Not only are most of them exquisitely beautiful, but the fit is indescribable. You truly can feel the difference. Of course I fully realize that most of us are not fortunate enough to have a closet full of Jimmy Choos and Manolo Blahniks, (my personal experience with them has been restricted to fashion shows) but it really is worth the investment to purchase the best quality you can afford. You will feel great about how you look, and your feet will be happy too.

For the final touch, I personally prefer a classic handbag, generally opting for good quality leather and nothing too trendy (although sometimes in a great color!) I think that handbags are just as much fun as shoes, if not more so. They give us such a wonderful way to accessorize and complete a look. And the nice thing about handbags—although there are plenty of fabulous designer bags out there, it isn't necessary to own one in order to look well put together. Beautiful handbags come in all price ranges. All you need to have is a good eye.

Wrapping it all up—when you are going shopping or considering what's in your closet, keep in mind the importance of dressing appropriately for your age, your lifestyle, and the occasion. Look for good quality, and remember that quality can be found in all price ranges. It doesn't necessarily have to be expensive, but it does have to be cut well and made of a good fabric.

Fashion changes, but style endures."

— Coco Chanel

PART TWO

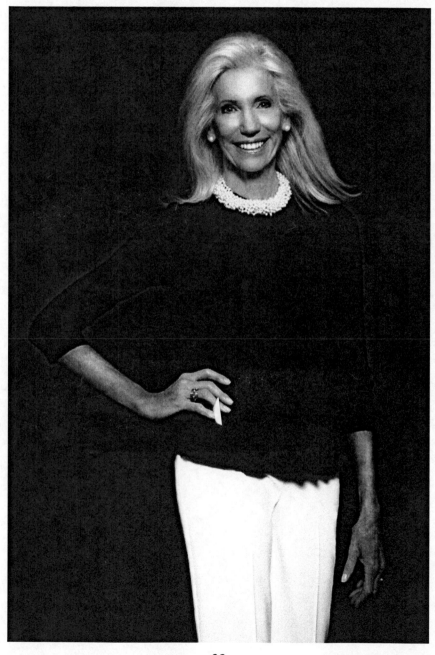

CHAPTER 10: So Now...What's next?

The best way to predict the future is to create it

— Abraham Lincoln

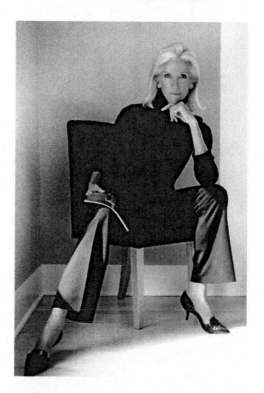

Looking Ahead

I love that quote—*"The best way to predict the future is to create it,"* because it says that we are each responsible for our own next chapters, and that it is up to us to go out and make it happen, whatever "it" is. It reminds us that we have to be proactive, and that means be willing to take the first action steps.

An action step may br something as simple as keeping our eyes and ears open to all of the possibilities and opportunities that are out there. Believe me, they exist all around us. The key is to be open to them, to keep our senses tuned into the world around us, and to be able to take an idea and run with it when the opportunity strikes.

Women stop me all the time looking for answers to "What's next? Where do I go from here?" Perhaps the nest has just emptied, a marriage or a relationship has ended, or they have become bored and restless with a career that once fulfilled them but no longer does. Whatever the reason, they have come to a major crossroads in their lives, and suddenly they have no idea which direction to take. In other words, we women have mid-life crises too.

I can empathize with their feelings of emptiness and uncertainty. I can understand it. I know what's it's like to feel that way, and I was determined not to let it happen to me. Let me tell you what I did and how I found my own "What's Next."

I had grown up, the only child of a very successful career woman who had broken through all the barriers against wives and mothers having careers outside the home by taking off to fly across the Andes on a business venture with the heads of Intercontinental Hotels and Pan American Airlines. IHC had just become the new subsidiary of Pan Am and they were eager to make the most of my mother's expertise, knowledge and connections in South America as they strategized the best locations to build their hotels.

I grew up knowing that as women we have other options beyond being housewives and mothers. Back in the '60's and '70's when our children were growing up, there was nothing I wanted more than to be at home with them. I considered being a good mother, being there for them, the most important job in the world. I believed that if Wally and I didn't do a good job raising our six children, nothing else that we did would matter. But I also knew that that phase of my life wouldn't last forever, that one day the children would grow up and take off on their own, and I would have many years stretching out ahead of me to fill. Even as I ice skated with them in the winter, rode the ferry boat out to Island Beach in the summer, or cooked meals for the family dinners we had every night, I knew that the day would come when all of that would end and it would be time to move on to something else. And so, as I went about these activities, as I read bedtime stories, baked cookies and gave splashy bubble baths, in the back of my mind I would think about the life I would pursue later on. I would think about what I wanted to do next.

Years later, when the children had all gone off to college and only the youngest remained at home, Wally was presented with a great opportunity. We had been going out to Carmel, California to visit my parents once or twice a year for many years, and he had developed a very nice relationship with the headmaster of the Stevenson School in Pebble Beach. One day in the spring of the late '80's he received an offer from Stevenson to do an exchange year with a faculty member from their English department. We would go to live in his house on the Pebble Beach campus and he would come and live in our house in Greenwich. Each would teach the other's classes. My mom had just been diagnosed with cancer and it was thought to be terminal. Knowing what a wonderful opportunity this would provide for me to be with her, and ready for a change after having been in Greenwich for twenty-five years, we grabbed it.

As we prepared for our year in California, I looked forward to moving to a whole new environment. After spending most of our lives on the East Coast, the idea of living on the magnificent Monterey Peninsula at the edge of the Pacific Ocean was more enticing than I can say. For so many years we had tuned into CBS-TV on snowy January afternoons to watch the AT&T Pebble Beach National Pro-Am, dreaming about how wonderful it would be to actually be there in the midst of all that beauty, but never believing that it would ever happen. Well—it did and we went for it! We embraced our new adventure with all of the enthusiasm and open-mindedness that one could imagine.

As it turned out, we never went back to Greenwich except to move. Wally fell right in with the Stevenson School, relishing everything about it, and so when he was offered a permanent position, he took it.

We enjoyed our first couple of years in California, going down to Big Sur and up to San Francisco as often as possible. During that time, we had three daughters living on the west coast, and it was Heaven having them close by. California had everything! It was so different from what we had been used to. We traveled to Lake Tahoe, Marin County, Palm Desert, Santa Barbara, San Francisco, the wine country and L.A. It was nice to have some time off to just be us, to explore our new home state and to have some time together. After a while, however, Wally's duties at Stevenson were keeping him increasingly busy, and I started getting restless. It was time to go out and create my own What's Next.

You gain strength, courage and confidence with every experience in which you really stop to look fear in the face. You must do the thing which you think you cannot do.

Eleanor Roosevelt

Someone had suggested that I might look into Pebble Beach Resorts for employment opportunities. The idea of venturing out into the world to see if I could make it in a corporate environment came as a real challenge, but I couldn't get it out of my mind. So although the idea initially filled me with fear (of not being qualified for anything,) after thinking about it, I thought, "Well, why not?" Our new life in California seemed like the perfect time to make the transition. The children were grown, and I knew it was My Time. At times the uncertainty was larger than the dream, but when fear and hesitation crept in, I immediately pushed them away and replaced them with the mental image of becoming the successful career woman I had envisioned.

I knew there were steps I would have to take in order to make all of this happen. I couldn't just wish for it. If you find yourself in a similar situation, this is my advice to you:

- Expand your skills. Get comfortable using a computer, if you aren't already.
- Learn how to use social network... FaceBook, Twitter, Instagram, Pinterest. These are all tools that will be of value in almost any job you seek.
- Go back to school if you want to advance yourself in a specialized field.
- Network! Network! Network! Join the Chamber of Commerce and other organizations in your area where

you will meet people who may fit into your future What's Next.

- Go out on informational interviews to learn more about an organization or business that interests you.

There were many moments when I stopped to remember Eleanor Roosevelt's famous words. Often I would have to push myself to move forward and "do the thing I thought I could not do"—like making that first visit to Pebble Beach's Human Resources Department - but I persevered—and won. And so can you. Let me tell you what happened.

CHAPTER 11: The Turning Point

*Ask for what you want. Ask for help, ask for input, ask
for advice and ideas—but never be afraid to ask.*

— Brian Tracy

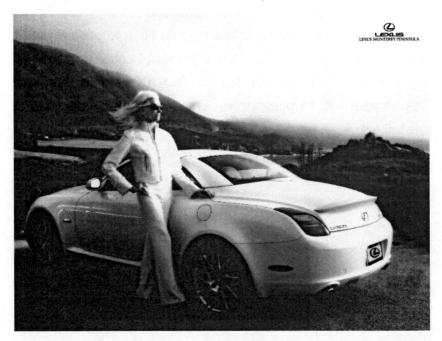

𝔉irst of all, remember that opportunities are all around us. If we keep our eyes and ears open, and are tuned into our surroundings, we can discover a world of possibilities for What's Next. What excites one person may be totally wrong for another, but believe me, there is something out there for all of us. Let me tell you about my experience.

As I just told you in the previous chapter, when we arrived on the Monterey Peninsula, I began thinking about the possibility of working at the iconic Pebble Beach Resorts; however, the idea of actually going over to their Human Resources Department and applying for a job terrified me. After all, I had minimal work experience, knew nothing about computers, and had never worked in the hospitality arena.

After much positive self-talk, however, and doing my homework on what exactly Pebble Beach Resorts was all about, I pushed myself out the door and took that first step. And that—the taking of the First Step—is how it all starts. Once you've done that, you're on your way.

As I said, I had nothing to offer Pebble Beach other than a fierce desire to work there, so (after three visits to the Human Resources Department) when they offered me a summer job in the pro shop with the college kids, I grabbed it. The important thing was to get my foot in the door. My advice to you if you are just starting out - Never mind your age. Never mind how entry level the job may be. Just get there and start doing it. During the few months that I worked in the pro shop, I took advantage of the opportunity to learn as much as I could about the Resorts and how they operated. I made friends with the people who worked there—people in sales and marketing, in catering and conference services, the guys in the golf division, the people in grounds keeping and housekeeping, the people in Pebble Beach's seven restaurants and those who worked at the spa, front desks and guest services. I talked to them all and listened carefully as they told me about what they did.

The other area I had to tackle was learning how to use a computer—an absolute necessity—so on my days off I went over to the Monterey Peninsula Community College and enrolled in a class. It was so much fun to conquer something new!

By the end of that summer, I had come a long way from when I first walked into the Human Resources Department and was ready to move on. When an administrative position opened up in the Marketing Department, I applied for it and got it.

The first few weeks were a little scary and certainly challenging, but with each day that went by, my knowledge and confidence grew. The following year I became an executive assistant and supported the senior vice president of marketing and the director of marketing. While I was doing this, I also had the opportunity to learn a lot about public relations because my good friend, Molly, who handled it, worked in the same office, and she frequently asked for my assistance in planning and executing special events and press trips. We did everything from credentialing media for the AT&T Pebble Beach National Pro-Am, to helping the USGA with the US Open Championships. We managed photo shoots and entertained the media, both on property and in New York and LA. It was great fun, and I knew that if Molly ever moved on to something else, I wanted to have that position.

One day, after I had been at Pebble Beach for four years, that day came, and when it did, I immediately went into my boss's office (the senior vice president of marketing) and asked for it. Much to my amazement, he looked at me, and then he said, "You've got it!" Lesson learned—Ask for what you want. You will be amazed at how often you get it.

OK—So now I had my dream job. I was the new public relations and media manager for the famed Pebble Beach Resorts; however, no sooner had I just gotten started than the unthinkable happened.

Assume that everything that happens to you does so for some good. All events contain an advantage for you - if you look for it

Picture this.... It was the first day of my brand new job, and I was responsible for a crew of one hundred that had come from LA to shoot print ads and commercials for Cadillac, the new brand partner of Pebble Beach. They were to be with me for a week, and they had a very lengthy shot list that included Pebble Beach Golf Links, 17-Mile Drive, the Beach & Tennis Club, the Spa, and the hotels. It was my responsibility to stage it all, make sure that they had everything they needed, and to be the liaison between the crew and the Resorts. That morning I had agreed to meet them on the seventh hole. It was 5:00 o'clock and it was still dark and slippery on the cart path. As I was running out to meet them,

I suddenly stumbled on the edge of the path, took a flying fall, landing hard on the ground, and ended up with a broken foot and a sprained ankle. All of this and I hadn't even met them yet!

Fortunately for me, a grounds keeper happened to be nearby and came right over to help me up and transport me the rest of the way to meet the crew. Smiling broadly and doing everything within my power to appear capable and confident, I arrived on the scene to greet them with warmth and enthusiasm and to assure them that despite the rocky start, this was going to be one heck of a successful shoot, and that both the client (Cadillac) and the Resorts would be thrilled with the results.

At that time, Cadillac had a campaign running set to that marvelous oldie, "Making Whoopee." One of the shots included a couple, all decked out in black tie, laughing and kidding around as they precariously walked along the edge of the pool at the Beach & Tennis Club. It was scripted so that all of a sudden, he gives her a little push from behind, and in she goes! Followed immediately by him. Splashes, smiles, hugs, kisses.... the music swells. End of scene. Happy client. Happy Pebble Beach.

Day 2 arrived. Bandaged and on crutches, I once again went out to meet my crew. The shoot was going well, we were on schedule, and they were getting exactly the shots they wanted. Just as I was starting to relax into the way the morning was progressing, my cell phone rang, and it was my doctor calling to tell me that the tests he had run the week before had come back positive and that I had uterine cancer—something both my mother and her mother had died from. He told me that he was scheduling surgery for the following week and asked that I come down to his office the next day for a pre-op workup.

Day 3 dawned, and once again and still on crutches, I had to leave my Cadillac crew and head for the doctor's office. As he put his stethoscope to my chest, a look of concern came over his face, and he told me that he was picking up an arrhythmia. He said he wasn't going to perform surgery until he had sent me to see a cardiologist, which he did that afternoon. As it turned out, I had a severe case of cardiomyopathy (weakened heart muscle) complicated by ventricular tachycardia—an arrhythmia that can put you into sudden cardiac arrest.

Now I was down three for three, and I truly felt as though the Universe was putting me to the test. The gauntlet had been thrown: To give up and back off from this demanding new job, or to say, "Hell no! I am going to beat this and go on to making the second half of my life even more phenomenal than the first half had been!" That is exactly what I did. Pebble Beach Resorts held my job for me while I had surgery for the cancer and a cardiac defibrillator implanted for the heart condition. A couple of months later I went back to work—stronger and better than ever. The lesson I learned here? Look at challenges as your greatest opportunities.

CHAPTER 12: Confidence—Be A Winner Before You Begin

Fear is a four-letter word. Feel the exhilaration of leaping into the unknown and tasting the sweet fruit of bravery. Taking the chance is its own reward.

— Valerie Ramsey

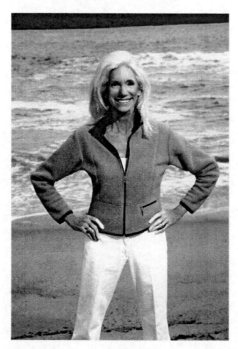

A can-do attitude is the key to thinking positively. There are times when it's important not to be afraid to take risks, whether it's a calculated risk or a gut feeling. When an opportunity comes along that feels right, even if it's something you've never done before, trust your instincts, think positively and say a resounding, "Yes!" Often times the details fall into place once you've taken that first leap of faith. When you have that feeling of jubilation when you're excited and something feels right, maybe tingly all over, then you know you're on track. It's your job to believe you can do it. After that you'll be rewarded and shown why going with your beliefs and gut feelings was the right thing to do. On the other hand, when your stomach doesn't feel right about something, that's your intuition telling your mind not to go forward. Women's intuition is a remarkable gift and when we are in tune with it, there isn't much we can't accomplish when we use our minds in conjunction with our feelings. It's all about confidence, and the more we test ourselves and move out of our comfort zones, the more confident we become.

Let me tell you a story to illustrate my point. I had never seriously thought about modeling. Oh sure—back when I was a teenager in boarding school, I would look at the pages of Glamour and Seventeen (a popular magazine in the 50's) and muse about what an exciting life it would be to travel to so many exotic locations and be photographed in such delicious looking clothes. My roommate and I even had a collage on our wall of pages torn from those magazines. But that was a daydream like many of us had when we were fifteen and sixteen. When I got into my twenties and thirties and had my family to take care of, in the back of my mind was the lure of a corporate career in the second half of my life that enticed me—not the idea of becoming a model.

Fast forward about forty years to the year 2002. By now I was sixty-three and had been in my public relations job for five years. I had gotten through those challenging first weeks when I had had to overcome both cancer and heart disease before I could move on, but I had succeeded, and the second half of my life was unfolding just as I had hoped. One day I was out on the golf course overseeing a photo shoot for a golf television special when the producer surprised me by saying, "You have a great look. You should be doing something with it. Let me take a few pictures and send them up to an agency in San Francisco. Let's see what happens." At first I resisted, thinking it was totally unrealistic that any modeling agency would be interested in a sixty-three year old woman, but he was persistent and so I eventually gave in.

Have you ever noticed that just when you least expect it, something amazing comes completely out of the blue and drops in your lap? Change can happen in a moment!

I have a favorite inspirational writer and speaker, Mike Dooley. His website is www.tut.com and on it you will find all sorts of positive, motivational thoughts and ideas that I promise you, will resonate and make your day. You can even get these marvelous quotes delivered daily to your email– a beautiful way to wake up. I would like to quote one of them here:

"If you were able to look back at your most brilliant successes, stunning comebacks, amazing catches, and smokin' ideas, and you were to find that virtually all of them seemed to materialize out of thin air, when you least expected them, and that they had exceeded even your greatest expectations at the time, how excited would you be about the new day?"

Well, that's exactly what happened. No sooner had the photos been sent to Stars the Agency in San Francisco than I received a phone call asking me if I would like to come up and sign a contract? Stunned—and full of trepidation about taking on the idea of photo shoots and catwalks—something in my gut told me to just do it. I listened to my intuition, and a few days later I was on my way to becoming a model. There was a caveat, however. I loved my PR job entirely too much to give it up, so I agreed to take on casting calls and modeling jobs only when my schedule permitted. Like so many things in life, it all worked out, and I entered a brand new world that I never could have imagined—well, at least not in the last fifty years!

It wasn't long before my confidence level was put to the test because a few weeks later I was booked to do a runway fashion show for the Boys & Girls Club of San Francisco in the Grand Ballroom of the Fairmont Hotel on top of Nob Hill. It was just before Christmas, and they were going to show fabulous ball gowns, evening clothes and jewelry from Wilkes Bashford (San Francisco's answer to Bergdorf Goodman in New York).

On the morning of the show, I arrived at the Fairmont and entered the ballroom. What I saw put fear into me like you wouldn't believe! There in front of me were big round tables for the twelve hundred guests who were to arrive, and a T-shaped runway of what seemed like enormous proportions. I had never done a runway show before and was quite overwhelmed by the thought of how in the world I was going to do this! I walked through the venue, taking it all in—the beautiful Christmas decorations and even Wilkes himself putting the finishing touches on the festive tables—and made my way backstage. There I found a scene that replicated some I'd seen in movies—a large hair and makeup station manned with a team from a salon on Maiden Lane—at the ready to transform us all into beautiful creatures ready to celebrate the holidays. What I saw next came as another surprise—something I wasn't prepared for. There were lots of models on hand—mostly young guys and girls roughly in the 18-22 age range—all running around in thongs and next-to-nothing undergarments getting fitted. They turned and looked at me—this silver haired older woman who had come into their midst—curiosity on their young faces. I laughed and blurted the first thing that popped into my head: "Kids, your den mother is here! This is my first runway show, and I am counting on you to get me through it.": They were wonderful. They greeted me enthusiastically and assured me that they would, and then one of the members from the hair and makeup team stepped forward and promised me that he would be there every time I went on or came off the runway, to "fluff" and encourage me. He was so kind. I will never forget what a difference he made to me that day.

At the end of the show, which was heavily choreographed to lively Christmas music, the most amazing thing happened. I actually got a standing ovation from the audience! As it turned out, they loved seeing an older model on the runway—someone they could relate to.

I had gotten through another challenge by visualizing a successful outcome. When I had first walked into that enormous ballroom, set up with tables for twelve hundred and an alarmingly long runway, I had been overcome with nerves. I had no choice, of course, but to forge ahead, and so I did exactly what I'm suggesting you do in a similar situation. I took a few deep breaths (it's impossible to feel nervous when you're deep breathing—did you know that? Try it!) and then I visualized myself walking down that runway with all the confidence of a seasoned super model. I visualized the way I would glide, turn, stop, and flawlessly glide back. By having a strong mental image of the great success I would have that day, I was able to overcome my fear and have an unforgettably positive experience.

Positive Thinking

What fascinates me is the knowledge and power of positive thinking that I've explored and have successfully used during the different phases of my life. None other than Deepak Chopra has pointed to research that says we have over 65,000 thoughts per day, and out of these 65,000 thoughts, nearly 95% of them are the exact thoughts that we generated the day before. Would you have guessed that you have that many thoughts a day? Let alone that you have had them before! I read this and wondered what percentage of these thoughts is positive rather than negative—having 65,000 positive thoughts sounds like a wonderful thing, while having 65,000 negative, recurring thoughts sounds absolutely awful. I've always been interested in the role our thoughts play in creating our lives; it's proven that through our minds the thoughts and words we create have the ability to create and shape our life experience.

Sometimes we'll hear or read a simple phrase that sticks in our mind. These phrases can form a strong belief that becomes our mantra. One of my favorite examples is, "Leap and the net will appear." I strongly believe that great success often involves taking a great risk. Jumping into my new public relations role at Pebble Beach felt very risky to me. It was a completely new venture, and although I felt confident that I could handle it, like anything new, it was rather frightening at first. As time went on, however, and new challenges were successfully met with every passing day, my confidence level grew. Every time I took on an assignment that called for something new, I immediately visualized a positive outcome and jumped in. Eleanor Roosevelt—you are one of my many heroes.

CHAPTER 13: Break Out Of The Old And Learn Something New

Learn something new. Try something different.
Convince yourself that you have no limits.

— Brian Tracy

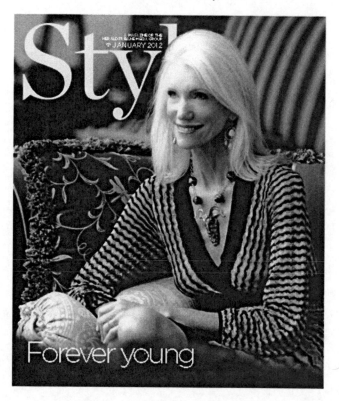

I decided to begin this chapter by revisiting and updating the chapter on trying something new from my first book because there is so much valuable information in it for the new reader. When was the last time you ventured out and learned something new? I don't mean reading the morning paper and learning a bit of trivia or the story behind the headline of a world event...I mean when was the last time you learned a new skill, craft or hobby? It used to be that by the time most people reached their thirties and forties, they had settled into a lifestyle or career that didn't require learning new skill sets. Or they had been so busy raising children they hadn't taken the time to continue to develop their own growth by consciously learning a new craft or skill. In recent decades, however, technology has boomed at such a rapid pace that we have all been forced to jump on the techno-train or be left behind at the station. I found this to be true after Wally and I faced an empty nest and moved to California. Once we were settled, I made the decision to start a career. The first thing I did was to sign up for computer classes. I remember walking in the first day and seeing all of those computers lined up in rows around the classroom. That was about twenty years ago, so you can imagine what the room looked like—clunky computers with even clunkier monitors. But as scary as the first sight of that room was, I was at the same time excited because I knew that that basic computer class would give me the confidence and technology exposure that I needed in order to land an administrative assistant position at Pebble Beach.

Technology is an easy example to fall back on because we've all had to face it—even if it's simply to send an email to family and friends or use a cell phone. There are so many interesting, challenging, and rewarding skills and hobbies to be learned depending on whether you're taking up a second career or wanting something new to do on the weekends.

For those of us who go through career changes late in the game, there are often obstacles that we have to move out of the way, step over, or face head on in order to achieve our goal. Some are a matter of societal influences, while others are a matter of educating ourselves further. These obstacles might include:

- Ageism
- Lack of credentials
- Lack of the appropriate degree (bachelors, masters, PhD, etc.)
- Lack of certification
- Reduced salary

- Lack of self-confidence
- Being told you're over qualified
- Lack of employment opportunities

The list above provides some of the excuses and barriers we can come up with to avoid change and growth. But they are just that—excuses. The less power you feed them, the smaller they become. Let's address these excuses for not trying something new.

Ageism

This one is easy for me to address simply because of my personal experience. I don't think many can argue with the fact that if I can get a job in the corporate world in my fifties or became a model in my sixties, there probably isn't much that anyone couldn't do if they put their mind to it. We are fortunate that our age group dominates much of the population and, therefore, we are able to support each other as we move into new fields and experiences. Many of the people I've worked with are baby-boomers themselves and are inspired by my story—and the stories of others just like me—because they, too, are making radical changes in their lives and can relate well to me. "Sixty is the New Forty" is the prevalent catch phrase, and if we're accepted as forty-year-olds, then why not take advantage of it?

And yet, sixty is still sixty—only it's a totally revamped sixty. Sixty isn't old anymore. Sixty is healthy, strong, sexy, vibrant, involved, curious, active, seeking to add new dimensions to our lives—in short—better than ever. We have much in common with the forty year olds, and yet we also have a tremendous advantage over them. We have maturity, life experience and confidence on our side. These attributes can take us a long way down the road to new successes. As long as we get out there and try!

Lack of credentials

In my case I came into the workforce after being a stay at home mom for nearly twenty-five years. On the surface, my credentials were diapers, bottles, home cooked meals, tying shoes and anything else you can think of when raising six children. But, on a deeper level, I had an innate ability to manage, to organize, and to deal with conflict. Go on any job interview and these three topics will surely come up. Even so, when I arrived in California, I took a computer class because I knew I needed it, and it gave me the credentials I needed on my resume to land the interview. Once I walked into the interview, the rest was up to me.

Lack of the appropriate degree:

There are cases where a degree is necessary to change careers. For example, my daughter, Heather, had been an office manager for fifteen years when she decided she wanted to be an English teacher. With only an associate's degree, she needed two more years of school to complete her bachelor's degree. Nowadays there are many schools offering degree programs for adults returning to school. She was fortunate to be living in Charlottesville, Virginia, and she discovered such a program at the University of Virginia. Within two years, she graduated from UVA with a Bachelors of Interdisciplinary Studies concentrating in English and secondary education. English classes dominated her coursework, and she went on to teach high school English for two years before taking the next step to become a full-time writer. She went back to school at the age of thirty-five and was younger than many of her classmates who were ten or twenty plus years older. She discovered that not only did earning her degree open doors that had previously been closed, but the experience of going back to school later in life was entirely different from the college experience she had when she was eighteen. Everyone she interacted with was excited and motivated to be back in school, and many of them had children of their own who were in college at the same time! Degree programs for adults are available both online and in classrooms, depending on the school and the curriculum.

Lack of certification

Degrees aren't always required. Thank goodness, because some of us don't want to write papers or sit in a classroom again! But, there are some exciting careers that do require at least a certification. For example, massage therapy, personal training, interior decorating, medical, dental, and many computer related fields require certifications. These programs vary in depth and venue but provide students with the certification and education needed to enter the field. Because they are much more specific than a liberal arts degree, the training is intense, and students come out of the programs thoroughly educated...assuming they've worked hard! These programs are a terrific way to meet people who have the same interest you do, and they might provide contacts you'll need later. It's a great opportunity to network!

"You're overqualified"

How many times have you heard someone say, "I went out on a job interview for something I really wanted, only to be told, 'You're overqualified?'" Particularly if that person has already been in the workforce for some time. Linda Ginac of the Ginac Group in Austin, TX has some excellent suggestions for confronting this issue.

- Be upfront about what appeals to you about the job.
- Use your accomplishments to show why you would be a good fit for that particular position.
- Don't allow salary to become an issue.
- Tell the interviewer that you're looking to extend the current skills that you have and to learning more as you apply them to the new position.
- Finally—offer to make a commitment that you will not leave the position for a year, two years, whatever seems right to you. That way an employer won't worry that you're only going to use the job to move on, or that you are a threat to him in his position.

Lack of self-confidence

"Self confidence" is an expression we hear throughout our lives. It is a term that defines us differently from one day to the next and from one experience to the next. When it comes to public relations, my self-confidence soars. However, when I was first asked to sit on a panel of speakers at San Jose State University, my self-confidence was questionable. This was my first foray into the realm of delivering an inspirational talk before a large gathering of people. Fortunately, once I was on stage it all fell into place, but the drive from Monterey to San Jose was another story! Self confidence comes from experience—the experience that only comes with age. As we master challenges, our confidence grows, and by the time we reach our fifties, we've experienced quite a bit. What I've found is that by taking a skill that we've mastered (for example, my modeling; or even my parenting), and applying it to a new experience, such as sitting on the panel at SJSU, I already had a leg up. I realized that the audience was inspired by my story. I used this as a connection to my modeling, which I was already comfortable with, drew on the familiar feelings of confidence in the modeling arena, and then applied it to my current seat on the panel. Talents are transferable. One experience overlaps another at times, and one can borrow from the other. Don't let a lack of self-confidence stop you from doing the things you really want to do.

***

Even though you won't find me learning to ski, there are definitely other adventures I'd be willing to try both before and after I retire. Different seasons will inspire new and different challenges, especially depending on where you live. Someone in the northeast or mountain areas just might be brave enough to take up skiing in their sixties, while others in colder regions could opt for cooking classes—what better place to be in the winter than in a warm kitchen learning new soup recipes! Alternatively, spring and summer would be a great time to join a gardening group, or a hiking club. Fall is a wonderful time to join a book club—hunkering down for cool weather reads—or a craft club just in time for the holidays or a second language class of a country you've always wanted to visit. The point being that every season brings new beginnings and fresh opportunities to delve into something new!

The trick to overcoming obstacles is to be connected to our thoughts and our actions. Once we overcome the fear of not being able to do something and start taking action toward accomplishing a goal, we see our dreams fall into place.

If it's a new hobby you're interested in learning, do some research online and locally to see if there are clubs or groups that meet. You can learn a lot from attending their gatherings, and most are informal with little or no pressure. Many local specialty stores have posters or mailings that announce classes and meetings. Stores that cater to cyclists might list a group ride that meets weekly. A running shop might be holding a clinic for beginning runners. Sewing shops are known for their classes and often have newsletters available by e-mail or snail mail. A store specializing in cooking ware might hold a monthly cooking class with different themes. At the coffee shop where Heather spends a lot of time writing, there is a woman who teaches a class in how to speak Italian, and most of her students are baby boomers with the intention of going to Italy. Additionally, there are many fliers on the bulletin boards of coffee shops and libraries that announce upcoming classes and interest groups. The opportunities are plentiful once you start to take notice of them.

On the internet, www.meetup.com is a wonderful place for finding local groups that cater to just about every hobby you can think of, including: hiking, cooking, writing, politics, language, knitting, scrapbooking, yoga, mediation, traveling, games, book clubs, poker and so many more. www.meetup.com is free to join and easy to use. If there's a group you want to start, you can do that too! As another option, look into the continuing education programs in your area. Many of them offer short classes in all sorts of different areas for reasonable prices. These are usually well attended and run a weekend or several weeks depending on the topic.

No matter what the new adventure you're considering is, take some time and jot down ideas in your. This is a great place to make lists as you write about what you want to accomplish. Use your journal to organize your plan of action, especially if it is on a larger scale such as going back to school. Write down a bulleted list of things you need to take care of before starting—phone calls or e-mails to potential programs, finances that need restructuring, time allotments, and anything else you can think of. The idea is to put pen to paper because doing so is like making a contract with yourself to make the dream happen. What you learn along the way will enrich you beyond anything you can possibly imagine.

Exercises for Learning Something New

Coming up with new ideas can feel overwhelming, making it easier to put the whole notion aside. I've come up with a few suggestions that might help jump-start your thinking -

Start with some reading material

What Should I do with My Life? By Po Bronson (Amazon) profiles dozens of people who make changes in their lives, primarily career. While this book is not a self-help book for changing careers, it provides anecdotes as examples and inspiration.

I Don't Know What I Want, But I Know It's Not This: A 12 Step Guide to Finding Gratifying Work by Julie Jansen (Amazon) is a favorite among readers who are in the midst of a career change and either need assistance in discovering what they want to do or if they simply need an encouraging nudge.

There are also a handful of books available such as *1000 Places to See Before You Die: A Traveler's Life List* by Patricia Schultz and *100 Things to Do Before You Die* by Neil Teplica that guide readers through events and places to visit. There might be something in one of these books that inspires you to take on a new hobby or adventure! At the very least these books motivate readers to experience new places.

Make your own list of things you want to do

Clear off the kitchen table and grab a notepad and pen. Once settled with a cup of coffee or tea, make a list of hobbies that you used to enjoy and haven't done in a while. If it's easier, go by decades—what did you really enjoy doing in your 20s that would still be of interest to you? The answers might surprise you! 30s? 40s? Did they involve crafts, sports, travel?

Next, consider things you always wanted to do, but didn't. Sometimes the resources may not have been available, or your family and career took priority. Revisit those ideas and add them to your list.

Television as an inspiration

Here's where you actually have permission to be a couch potato! Between the Home and Garden channels, Animal Planet, the Travel Channel, National Geographic, and many others, ideas are almost limitless. These stations have a myriad of programs that address just about any hobby, and for visual learners, they do a good job of providing step-by-step progress right on the screen. If you find a hobby of interest, you can follow up with internet searches or books for more details.

Don't go it alone

Involve your spouse or a girlfriend! Sign up for a weekend workshop. Lots of the ideas are co-ed and there are many that would appeal to both men and women alike. Women, particularly older women, embarking on something new can be powerful allies and can really inspire each other to stick with it. Besides, it's so much more fun to have a partner or a friend along than to take on something new by yourself.

Home Depot offers many free classes—who knows what home improvements might come of that! Along the same line, take your Home Depot learned skills and volunteer for Habitat for Humanity for a weekend. That's a wonderful way to give back to communities by helping people, and you'll meet interesting people with a joint cause.

Alternatively, find a local studio that offers glass blowing classes. The arts are therapeutic and fun. Something like glass blowing would be a great creative release, while still masculine in tone.

About town

Keep an eye out for happenings about town. Pull out the local paper, especially the weeklies that provide events, and circle anything that looks interesting. Run the ideas by your spouse or a friend and make a date of it. Additionally, pause and read the fliers on bulletin boards. Something might catch your attention.

Revisiting old hobbies rejuvenates the spirit. The ones we packed away might have been stored temporarily or for a long while, but like all treasures, their purpose is worth recapturing. Whether you go it alone, with your spouse, or with a friend, trying something new enriches your life and adds a dimension of happiness and excitement to those treasures that were boxed up and stored in your attic.

CHAPTER 14: Breaking Into Modeling: The Real Skinny!

'Fashion is not necessarily about labels. It's not about brands. It's about something else that comes from within you."

— Ralph Lauren *Ralph Lauren, 2008 runway show*

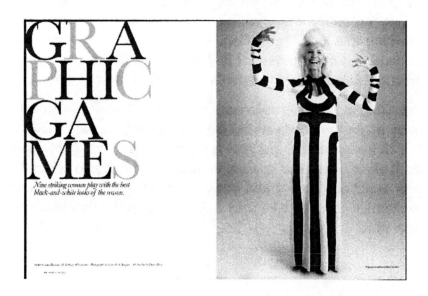

Because I'm often asked by both men and women who are interested in modeling and breaking into the industry, I wanted to share advice and information given to me by one of the top agents in the field, Susan Schwabinger, owner of Alexa Models & Talent in Tampa, FL.

Q. Your agency books jobs both nationally and internationally. What is your advice for someone wanting to break into modeling?

A. My advice is that you do not go out and have professional photos taken before meeting with an agent. In general, the photos will not work for the agency's marketing purposes and will only be a waste of time and money. Digital snapshots are sufficient to get you seen. Get a friend to take some photos for you... take these snapshots outside in natural light with very little makeup on, maybe just some mascara and lip gloss, because the agencies want to see how you photograph. Mix it up with some close ups of the face at different angles, some smiling so they can see your teeth, then I suggest a full length body shot that shows your figure and what kind of shape you're in. Once you have snapshots, be true to yourself and go with your intuition to see if the agency sounds right for you. When you go into an open call or have an appointment with an agency, they can generally tell right away if you would be a good fit or not. They won't want to take you on if they don't feel that they can market you.

One other piece of advice—be prepared for rejection. There will be a lot. Not every agency will have the right need for your look, so you may be turned down quite a bit. If this is not the right business for you, do not take it personally. This is a very selective industry, and only a small percentage of people will be able to successfully support themselves in this line of work.

Q. Should a model be represented by more than one agency?

A . A model in most cases should have ONLY 1 AGENCY PER MARKET. So, you can have an agent in LA, Chicago, Dallas, NYC etc. but generally not within a fifty-mile radius of the agency you first sign with (known in the business as your "mother agency.") In a "Lifestyle" situation, models may be allowed to have more than one agent. That should be discussed with the agent you are signing with. It is a case-by-case situation.

Q. How do you see the demand for baby boomer models? What is the industry looking for and how much work is there, really?

A. The demand for older models is definitely increasing. Baby boomers are living longer, they are more vibrant and healthy at an older age, and consequently that's opening up a whole new market for advertising. Although this new generation of consumers is older, they do not consider themselves older. As we are clearly seeing, 60 is the new 40. Women specifically are buying millions of dollars' worth of products for anti-aging, and advertisers know that consumers are not going to want to buy them from younger models. There is a certain level of maturity and confidence that comes with women over 40, an elevated level they bring to the marketplace. Consequently, advertisers want a model who is going to be a good representative for their product. They're looking for people who are attractive and whom the general population can relate to and have confidence in. It is important to note, too, that the baby boomers are the ones with the money now. With that in mind, the advertisers are formulating new strategies to sell to this demographic.

One other good thing to remember when you do sign with an agency is that they are working for you—not the other way around. As models we sometimes tend to forget that.

Q. Are the newspaper ads seeking models legitimate? How do you tell if it's legitimate or isn't?

A. Modeling agencies NEVER EVER advertise in the newspaper. Or advertise anywhere. They may put a type of model needed, babies, for example out via Social Media Websites, such as Facebook, Twitter, etc., but if they were looking for a particular type of model, it would be within their own networking channels.

 Q. Do you recommend runway, print or commercials for breaking in?

A. There is no particular area of modeling to "break" into. Runway-requires a very specific model type and body type. There are height requirements, measurement requirements and most of all "THE WALK".

Commercials - Once again - very specific to the BRAND of the product and what the demographics are that they are selling to. For example, the models in a Wendy's commercial would not be the same models that you would see in a fragrance commercial or a pharmaceutical commercial.

Print- Once again, there are all different types of models....you have lifestyle, editorial and catalogue.

A shorter model will be able to do commercials, although they will not be able to do runway modeling, catalogue and some print.

So there is NOT any real definitive area for a model to start in. It all depends on the type of model that you are.

The bottom line....Anyone who has an inkling that modeling is something she'd like to investigate to see if it's right for them, I think by all means go for it. You never know until you try!

CHAPTER 15: When Life Hands You An Audition, Give It Everything You've Got

It's never too late to be who you might have been

— George Eliot

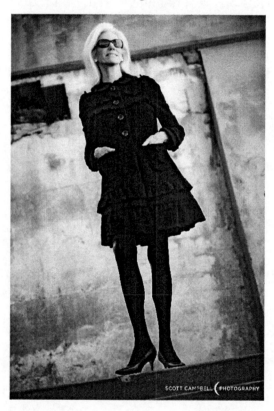

*Y*ou just never know when an amazing opportunity is going to seemingly come out of nowhere. About a month after the Monterey Herald piece came out, I had a phone call at work from Peter Greenburg, who was then the travel editor for The TODAY Show. I hadn't met Peter in person, but we had become telephone friends because of my work at Pebble Beach. Peter was calling to tell me that Jim Bell, the executive producer of TODAY, was traveling in California with his wife, four little boys and their nanny. They were headed down the coast from San Francisco to L.A. and wanted to have a stopover in Pebble Beach. Could we take care of them? Needless to say, I jumped right on it and arrangements were made. That evening I was at an event off property, but knowing that Jim and his family would be going in to have dinner at Roy's Restaurant at The Inn at Spanish Bay, where they were staying, I didn't want to lose the opportunity to shake his hand and meet him in person, so I left the event I was attending and headed back to Spanish Bay. Jim and his delightful family arrived right on schedule, and we were able to chat for a few minutes. He was extremely personable and nice, and his family was beautiful. I was so glad I had taken the opportunity to meet them.

I didn't let it end there, however. This was an "audition" that I recognized and wanted to make the most of. So when Jim got back to New York, I took a copy of the newspaper article, put it in a FedEx envelope, and attached a note saying, "I'm sending you this on the chance that it might fit in with a story line you have coming up." As it turned out, it did. I had a lovely email back from him immediately telling me that my timing was perfect and to stand by for a phone call from one of his producers.

About a week later I arrived at my desk to find a voicemail waiting from a TODAY Show producer asking me to call her. They were putting together a segment that would have Gail Sheehy and Racquel Welch in the studio discussing Gail's new book, *Sex and the Seasoned Woman*. In it, she focused on women who lived the second half of their lives with purpose and passion. TODAY felt that I exemplified that woman. The producer asked if I had a photo shoot coming up any time soon? They wanted to send a crew out to film the shoot, and then to spend a second day interviewing me at The Lodge where both my PR and modeling careers had begun. As it turned out, I did have a shoot on the books for Lexus down by Big Sur, and so arrangements were made. It turned out to be a wonderful segment, the whole experience being so much more than anything I could have ever imagined happening. All because I recognized an opportunity for an "audition" and went for it.

That wasn't the end of the story, however, and this struck me as even more funny than anything. A couple of months later when I was getting ready to leave for work, my cell phone rang, and it was another TODAY producer calling from New York to say that they were doing a segment on women who let their hair go gray. They remembered my silver hair from the first time I'd been on the show, and they wanted to know if I would come to New York to be on the show again and to talk about it? At first I was incredulous; they actually wanted to fly me to New York to talk about my hair! But they were quite serious, and so Wally and I went. What an unforgettable time we had! The other two guests on the show with me that day were Nora Ephron (*Sleepless in Seattle, You've Got Mail, I Feel Bad About My Neck*, and many other screenplays and books) and Christine Ebersole, who was staring on Broadway at the time. Ann Curry and Hoda Kotbe interviewed us, and we had a grand time. (By the way, Ann Curry is one of the kindest, nicest people you could ever hope to meet, and Hoda is out-of-this-world fabulous! I adore both of these amazing women).

Because of a lovely relationship I had with Tiffany's in Carmel (as a friend of the staff's—not as one of their top ten customers!) the New York Tiffany's invited me to come into their store on Fifth Ave & 57th Street to pick out anything I wanted to wear on TODAY. What fun to browse the store! I selected some incredibly wonderful Paloma Picasso pieces—a girl's dream come true! And best of all—after the show, when Wally and I went to return the jewelry to the store, they invited us up to their top floor where their team of European and Asian craftsmen were creating some of the fabulous brooches and other pieces we had seen downstairs. They showed us the entire intricate process—one that typically takes several months from beginning to end. It was fascinating—and such a rare treat to get a behind-the-scenes look at this iconic store.

All because of two things....my naturally silver hair! (Who would have ever guessed?) and because I recognized an opportunity and grabbed it. The lesson here—opportunities are out there. They can appear out of nowhere, when you least expect them, but if you keep your eyes and ears open, and your senses tuned in to your surroundings, anything can happen.

Grab a risk, and you won't be sorry for a might have been.

Arthur Mitchell Ransome

CHAPTER 16: Public Speaking—
When A New Opportunity Is
More Frightening Than Enticing

It is not failure itself that holds you back: it is the fear of failure that paralyzes you.

— Brian Tracy

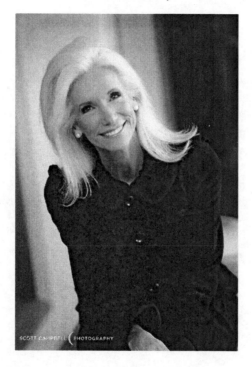

𝒟id you ever have a new opportunity come along that really

sparked your interest but at the same time terrified you? Something that sounded very tempting, that you knew you would love to do, but that you were scared to death you couldn't pull it off? It seems that my life has been full of these kinds of opportunities, some of which I've already told you about. Here is another experience I'd like to share with you because I think it could be of value.

We have all heard that the number one fear people have is the fear of public speaking. It even beats out fear of dying. Well, shortly after *Gracefully* came out, I had a phone call from Medtronic Corporation. They make many different types of medical devices including pace makers and implanted cardiac defibrillators. I had had two of their devices - first a Reveal monitor, (which was like an implanted EKG machine) and then a cardiac defibrillator. They were calling to tell me that they were putting on a Sudden Cardiac Arrest Leadership Conference co-hosted with the National Medical Association in Washington DC and to ask if I would be willing to go to Washington to address several hundred cardiologists? They wanted me to tell them as a lay person about my experience with viral cardiomyopathy and ventricular tachycardia? I had never spoken in public before at anything remotely like that, and at first the idea filled me with terror; however, I recognized two new opportunities when they called me. Most importantly, I knew that by complying with their request, I could be doing a lot of good by speaking to these world-renowned doctors about my own personal experience. And secondly—I saw this as a challenge that if successfully met, could move me past my fear of speaking in public. That idea greatly appealed to me because looking ahead I saw a world of opportunities to motivate and inspire others to create their own What's Next, just as I had. I told Medtronic that I would do it, and it turned out to be one of the best decisions I have ever made. The doctors who had gathered for the conference were so appreciative, and they made it known how glad they were that I had come to speak to them. That was all it took—the realization that my audience was behind me and that they truly cared about what I had to say. As soon as I realized that, there was nothing to be afraid of.

That conference turned out to be a valuable lesson for me in so many ways. The first thing I did when I found out I was going to be speaking was to buy a copy of Lee Glickstein's book, *Be Heard Now*. It is packed full of the best information you can imagine on getting over your fear of speaking in public. It's all about what he calls, "Transformational Speaking," making "soft" eye contact and listening to your audience with your heart. He calls it the "key ingredient in successful relationships, business skills such as management and team building, and all good communication." That book has become my Bible, and it is available from Amazon. You will never be fearful of speaking again after you have read it.

Tips For Easier Public Speaking

- Arrive early
- Personally greet as many people ahead of time as possible. You are establishing a rapport with them before you even get started.
- When you walk out to the podium, be still for a moment, smile, take a deep breath, and relax into the moment.
- Focus your attention on your audience, not on yourself.
- "Listen" to them, feel their support. Once you can do that with one audience, you can do it with any audience.
- Forget the customary greeting—Hello, I am so happy to be here..... Instead, jump right in with a great story that pertains to what you are there to talk about. This grabs their attention right off the bat. You can save your thanks for the end.

- Make eye contact with individuals in the audience and linger with each person for a few seconds while you are speaking
- Remember to pause. Don't race through your speech.
- Be humorous, particularly at yourself. This will make you human and endear you to your audience.
- Do your homework. Learn as much as you can about the company and the audience that you will be addressing; learn the names of the key players and use them in your speech
- Remember—they want you to succeed!
- If you can, open up the floor to a Q & A at the end of your speech. I love having this connection with an audience after I've finished speaking.
- If you have the time, stay for a while afterwards to greet and take more personal comments and questions.

I can promise you that taking this kind of opportunity and running with it can turn out to be one of the best things you ever did for yourself. You will be so gratified by the wonderful people that you meet, you will feel so good about sharing yourself with them and giving them something of value to take away, and best of all—you will have overcome one of the greatest fears that any of us faces.

One final thought—you never know who will be sitting in the audience that day. I have made some pretty amazing contacts when I have gone out to speak. You can too!

CHAPTER 17: Recognizing Life's Invitations

When Life opens a door right in front of you, walk through

— Mike Dooley

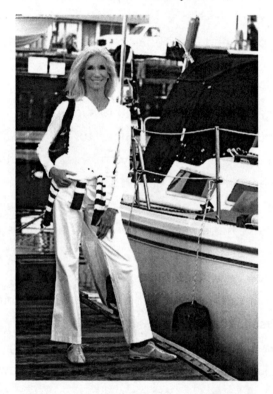

One day I had a phone call from a writer at the Monterey County Herald. I had just signed a modeling contract with Stars Agency in San Francisco, and Brenda Moore in the paper's features department thought it was a story that their readers would be interested in.... "63 year old grandmother becomes model." I was not nearly as enthusiastic about seeing my story in print as she was, but she persevered, and eventually I agreed. As it turned out, Brenda did a wonderful job, and before I knew what had happened, I discovered that her feature had been picked up off the national newswires and had started appearing in papers all across the country. As it popped up in cities like Boston, Chicago, Miami, L.A. and New York, I began getting the loveliest emails from men and women in city after city telling me how inspired they had been by my story. They wrote me about how they were in their fifties or sixties and had started to think that they were too old to have a new career or to pursue some other lifelong dream that they had put aside. After reading about how I had transitioned through staying at home with our children, into the corporate world, and then at sixty-three into modeling (while still maintaining my Pebble Beach PR career), they realized that if I could make these transitions in my 50's and 60's, they could too.

I would call my daughter, Heather Hummel, who is a writer, and I would read her these wonderful emails that were coming in almost every day. She soon recognized an opportunity to do something very worthwhile with them and suggested that we write a book. With her guidance, writing skills, and knowledge of the publishing world, we quickly landed the outstanding literary team of Whimsy, LLC. The next order of business was to finish writing the proposal, and once that was done, our agents, Olga Vezeris and Jackie Meyer, began shopping it to the top publishers in New York. *Gracefully—Looking and Being Your Best at Any Age* was quickly picked up by McGraw Hill, and once that happened, we concentrated on finishing the manuscript within the next seven months. *Gracefully* came out in the spring of 2008.

We wanted very much to have a celebrity write the foreword—someone who would be a perfect fit for the book and who lived her life in much the same way that I so whole-heartedly endorsed in the book. As I thought about it, Susan Lucci quickly came to mind.

I had had the great pleasure of meeting Susan and her husband, Helmut, a few months before when they came out to Pebble Beach as my guests. We had just opened the beautiful new Spa at Pebble Beach and the small, very elegant boutique hotel right next to it, Casa Palmero, and Entertainment Tonight had agreed to come up and film a segment on it with Susan. It took some doing with Susan's busy schedule, but we got her there and had an extraordinary four days. Susan did a gorgeous piece for ET at The Spa, the Beach & Tennis Club, and on the Bagpiper Terrace at The Inn at Spanish Bay while Helmut played golf to his heart's content. My husband, Wally, and I had the great pleasure of going out to dinner with Susan and Helmut and Paul and Cyndy Spengler of Pebble Beach twice while they were there. Paul was the Executive Vice President of Golf, and he and his wife, Cyndy, had been instrumental in helping me get Susan to come out. As it turned out, the couple had such a great time that they ended up spending an extra day!

I cannot end the story there without saying that Susan Lucci is without a doubt the sweetest, nicest, most down to earth person you could ever hope to meet. She is a brilliantly talented actress and businesswoman, and when someone is described as being "as beautiful on the inside as they are on the outside," that truly describes Susan. As I thought about whom to ask to write the foreword for us, when Susan came to mind, I called her and she most graciously said that she would be happy to do it.

That is an example of what can happen when we are open to new opportunities, even those that we don't recognize as being opportunities when they first come along. I never ever imagined Brenda Moore's article going any farther than the Monterey Peninsula, and yet it did, and that one event entirely changed my life.

Lesson learned—Change can happen in an instant, often when we least expect it. So when you get the chance—go for it!

CHAPTER 18: Sometimes It Takes A Team

In union there is strength

☐— Aesop

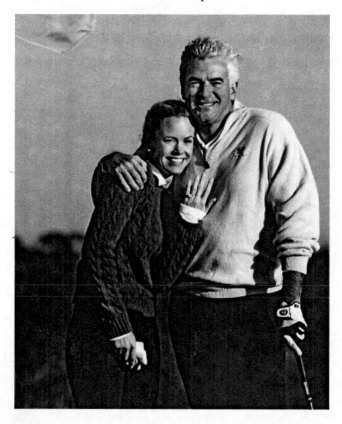

When I hit that roadblock of being diagnosed with both cardiomyopathy and cancer at the very start of my career, there was really never any doubt in my mind about the direction I was going to take. During the time I was going through surgeries and recovering, I was asked over and over again if I was sure that I wanted to go back to work—if I was certain that taking on this enormous public relations position was the right thing to do? Pebble Beach Resorts, after all, is so much more than just the golf links—iconic and beautiful as they are. The Resorts are also comprised of three other golf courses, three hotels, 17-Mile Drive, a spa, and seven restaurants. It hosts two major events each year—the Pebble Beach AT&T National Pro-Am and the Concours d'Elegance—and several smaller ones. In addition, it has also hosted five U.S. Open Golf Championships. Being the on-site public relations manager for all of this was an enormous undertaking, even with the outside help of Murphy O'Brien Communications in L.A. The responsibility was great. My hesitation was not. I had worked hard to achieve this dream. This was my What's Next and I wasn't about to let go of it!

I've told you about my decision to find a career and about my first week on the job, the turning point, and I've told you all about being "discovered" for modeling and my first big runway fashion show in San Francisco—about walking into the grand ballroom at the Fairmont Hotel and seeing it all set up to accommodate twelve hundred guests and how I visualized a successful outcome in order to get through that rather frightening new challenge.

I had had a goal and I had taken the first steps towards seeing it through. Thoughts. Words. Action. That is how you achieve What's Next. Let me tell you a few more important things that I learned because please remember—creating the second chapter of my life was just as untried and new to me as I'm guessing it is for some of you. Actually, as it turned out, it was the next two chapters!

What I want to write about now is the value of teamwork.

We can accomplish so much more when we work together. When we are searching for What's Next, we can often feel that we are alone, but once we set off on our new path, if we can get others on board with us, we become stronger and miracles can happen.

Going back to the fifteen years I was at Pebble Beach—from the time I was fifty-three until I was sixty-eight—it seemed that one new experience kept coming on the heels of another. I had already gone out and learned how to use a computer, so that was one big step in the right direction. The next was becoming familiar with all of the varied departments within the Resorts. There were eighteen hundred employees to keep everything running smoothly, and I came to know most of them, at least by face, if not always by name. In many cases they also became new friends.

I had to learn quickly how to be fast and efficient in taking on all of my new responsibilities. That meant becoming familiar with the many different departments—sales, catering/conference services, the front desks, food & beverage, the spa, golf, housekeeping, accounting, engineering, and resource management—because my job entailed interacting with all of them. A resort's reputation for excellence depends heavily on the teamwork of its employees. I loved this part of what I did. To me, working together with all of these great people to make something happen was one of the most enjoyable parts of my job. I was unfailingly impressed with both the professionalism and the friendliness that surrounded me. It was fun too! Let me give you one hilarious example of the teamwork that went on all the time.

One day in the early fall I received a call from a wonderful friend, Lisa Mesloh. Lisa and I had met a few years prior when she was with The Golf Channel and we were working on a promotion together. Lisa was (and is) a beautiful young blonde, smart and classy. We became instant friends the first time we met, and I've loved her ever since. She was calling to tell me that she had been dating someone whom I also knew, John O'Hurley, of Seinfeld (he played Peterman) and Broadway fame. Actually John has a long list of credits. He is a very talented man. John and I met when he was filming a very funny series for USA Network based on the courses that the PGA Tour was scheduled to play that year, and of course, Pebble Beach was one of them.

Lisa was calling to say that she and John were planning a golfing weekend to Pebble Beach to celebrate his birthday. She wanted to surprise him with a very special romantic dinner—something for just the two of them—and could I help her with the arrangements? Of course I could! Together we started talking about having Club XIX cater a beautiful cozy dinner in the wood paneled library at Casa Palmero, complete with the fireplace lit, candlelight, soft music and fragrant flowers. John would love it!

So fast forward a few days. The phone on my desk rang again, only this time it was John looking for my help. When they came up for the weekend, he wanted to surprise Lisa by proposing to her on the famed seventh hole. His idea was to have the engagement ring hidden in the cup, and not only did he want to surprise her, he also wanted photographers there to document it so that they could share the story with her family afterwards! She was not to suspect a thing, of course. Could I arrange that? Well—with the help of my fabulous Pebble Beach team, yes I could.

In the coming days plans were made, phone calls exchanged (although sometimes it was a little tricky keeping the two cell phone numbers and two sets of surprise plans separated) and the time for their arrival drew closer. Arrangements were made with the management team from Casa Palmero, the food & beverage team from Club XIX, the floral department, and the golf division. I called on Tom O'Neal and Gary Geiger, two of the greatest photographers in the world who do a lot of work for Pebble Beach, and explained to them what we wanted to do. They were into it immediately, suggesting that we "stage" the shoot as if for a golf layout. They would even bring an assistant, dressed as our "model," and the story when John and Lisa approached the seventh hole would be that they were shooting a print ad—they would step aside while our couple played through (but all the while quietly taking photographs)– and then they would resume their "shoot."

Well, John and Lisa arrived at Pebble Beach and checked in at Casa Palmero, where the staff was waiting on full alert and ready to carry off the plan. The photographers were well out of sight as the couple walked into the lobby. John surreptitiously handed off the ring box to the manager who slipped it into her pocket and a short time later got it into the hands of Tom and Gary.

It was late in the day, a beautiful, typical October afternoon.... bright and sunny but also very windy. Both John and Lisa are excellent golfers, and she also happens to be very competitive, so when he suggested a quick ride out to the famous par 3 seventh hole for a little friendly competition to see who could hit the lowest score on it, she agreed immediately. Meanwhile, the manager from Club XIX and his staff were arriving at Casa Palmero with the florist and her team to start turning the lovely little library into a romantic retreat for the birthday dinner, while Tom and Gary raced out to the seventh hole with the ring box to hide it in the cup and set up their equipment.

When John and Lisa arrived at the tee box, Lisa was ready for the challenge. With a 3 handicap, she was sure she could beat John hands down on this one. This is the iconic hole that I'm sure you've seen photos of and would recognize in an instant. The tee box sits up on a bluff, and a short distance below the green juts out into the ocean, surrounded by water on three sides. Remember when I said it was windy? Oh my goodness—was it ever—and just as Lisa took her drive off the tee box, a great gust blew in, carrying her ball over the green and into a sand trap. Next came John's turn. As they say, timing is everything, and as he teed off the wind died down again, allowing his ball to land in perfect position on the green. Now Lisa was down in the sand trap, getting ready to chip the ball up onto the green, but once again, luck was not with her as a second gust of wind carried it well beyond its target and into a bunker on the other side. When John easily knocked his ball into the cup, she was trying to be a good sport about it, but she was less than happy. Irritated with the way the strong wind was playing havoc with her shots, she called over to John to please pull the pin. As he did so, the corner of the wooden box was seen sticking up out of the hole—not the typical little blue box from Tiffany's, but a rosewood box that was larger than most ring boxes and slightly too large for the cup. Well—seeing this interference with her shot was the last straw for Lisa. Tossing her club down, she marched over to the offending box, yanked it out of the cup with a, "Would you look at that? There's something jammed in the darn hole!!!" and without even looking at it, hurled it towards the ocean. Horrified, and panicked that his magnificent diamond was about to disappear into Carmel Bay, John lunged towards the box and retrieved it just as it was rolling down the embankment. Snatching it up, he breathlessly ran back to where Lisa was standing on the green, threw himself down on his knee, took her hand, and said, "You don't understand. This is for you. I love you. I want to spend the rest of my life with you. Will you marry me?"

Naturally her reaction was the same as what any of ours would have been too—she burst into tears and shouted, "Yes!!!!!" Cameras were clicking, hugs exchanged, and an unforgettable moment had been perfectly documented. The happy ending to the story, as you can imagine, was the newly engaged couple hopping into their cart and heading back to Casa Palmero where, you guessed it, it was Lisa's turn to surprise John with his romantic birthday dinner.

None of this could have happened without teamwork. Whatever you might end up doing, wherever you might work, it is always so much better when you do it with a generous open mind, as an enthusiastic member of the team. Remember that your job is not an isolated one. You are part of a group whose purpose is to help your guest, your client, your customer, whomever. Put politics and the organization aside and just focus on being the very best team player that you can possibly be. You'll have a great time, and the rest of the team will love you for it.

By the way—this story played out so beautifully and had such a happy ending that for a long time afterwards, John used it as part of his opening act in Las Vegas.

More Of My Favorite Quotes

I believe in pink. I believe that laughing is the best calorie burner. I believe in kissing, kissing a lot. I believe in being strong when everything seems to be going wrong. I believe that happy girls are the prettiest girls. I believe that tomorrow is another day and I believe in miracles.

— Audrey Hepburn

Outer beauty attracts, but inner beauty captivates.

— Kate Angell, Squeeze Play

Beauty is not in the face; beauty is a light in the heart.

— Kahlil Gibran

The only real elegance is in the mind; if you've got that, the rest really comes from it.

— Diana Vreeland

A vigorous five-mile walk will do more good for an unhappy but otherwise healthy adult than all the medicine and psychology in the world.

— Paul Dudley White

Engagement Is Essential To Successful Aging.

— Gail Sheehy

Life is not about how many breaths we take, but how many moments take our breath away.

— Anonymous

To keep the body in good health is a duty, otherwise we shall not be able to keep our mind strong and clear.

— Buddah

Being deeply loved by someone gives you strength while loving someone deeply gives you courage.

— Lao Tzu

Against the assault of laughter nothing can stand.

— Mark Twain

Dwelling on the unimportant, stressing on the unintended, and freaking over the unknown, simply doesn't work... and are a bit like lighting a match in a dark room to make sure no one accidentally sprinkled any gunpowder on your bicycle, kept under the stairs, near the back porch in January.

— Mike Dooley

The only thing that makes the difference in the way you feel right now is the thought that you are thinking right now.

— Unknown

Be so happy that when others look at you, they become happy too.

— Yogi Bhaja

Do more than belong: participate

Do more than care: help

Do more than believe: practice

Do more than be fair: be kind

Do more than forgive: forget

Do more than dream: work

— William Arthur Ward

Confidence is courage at ease.

— Daniel Maher

The higher your energy level, the more efficient your body. The more efficient your body, the better you feel and the more you will use your talent to produce outstanding results.

— Tony Robbins

Do your homework, be prepared, and then go forward with a confident and positive spirit.

— Valerie Ramsey, *Gracefully*

Don't fret. It will happen differently anyway.

— Dutch saying

If you tackle it with humor and grace, you can pull off just about anything.

— Valerie Ramsey, *Gracefully*

The main reason someone moves mountains, wins friends, influences people, amasses a fortune, or anything else, is because they thought they would.

— Mike Dooley

No one would have ever crossed the ocean if he could have gotten off the ship in the storm.

— Charles F Ketterling

Dreams are renewable. No matter what our age or condition, there are still untapped possibilities within us and new beauty waiting to be born.

— Dr. Dale Turner

If you only look at what is, you might never attain what could be.

— Anonymous

Let me tell you the secret that has led me to my goal. My strength lies solely in my tenacity.

— Louis Pasteur

Whether you believe you can do a thing or not, you are right either way.

— Henry Ford

Optimism is the one quality more associated with success and happiness than any other.

— Brian Tracy

One of the most courageous things you can do is identify yourself, know who you are, what you believe in and where you want to go.

— Sheila Murray Bethel

Always go with the choice that scares you the most, because that's the one that is going to require the most from you.

— Caroline Myss

Do you really want to look back on your life and see how wonderful it could have been had you not been afraid to live it?

— Caroline Myss

The most common way people give up their power is by thinking they don't have any.

— Alice Walker

A beautiful woman used her lips for truth, her voice for kindness, her ears for compassion, her hands for charity and her heart for love. For those who do not like her, she uses Prayer.

— Unknown

Life should NOT be a journey to the grave with the intention of arriving safely in an attractive and well-preserved body, but rather to skid in sideways - Chardonnay in one hand - chocolate in the other - body thoroughly used up, totally worn out and screaming "WOO-HOO, what a ride!"

— Hunter S. Thompson

And Finally

Life is short, break the rules, forgive quickly, kiss slowly, live truly, laugh uncontrollably, and never regret anything that made you smile. Twenty years from now you will be more disappointed by the things you didn't do than by the ones you did. So throw off the bowlines. Sail away from the safe harbor. Catch the trade winds in your sails. Explore. Dream. Discover.

— Mark Twain

Alfred Lord Tennyson's "Ulysses"

It may be that the gulfs will wash us down;

It may be we shall touch the Happy Isles,

And though we are not now that strength which in old days

Moved earth and heaven, that which we are, we are—

Made weak by time and fate, but strong in will;

To strive, to seek, to find, and not to yield

What the poem is saying is that while it's tempting to play it safe, the more we're willing to risk, the more alive we are. In the end, what we regret most are the chances we never took.

I HOPE YOU DANCE

Lee Ann Womack Songwriters: Sillers/Sanders

Whenever one door closes I hope one more opens
Promise me that you'll give faith a fighting chance
And when you get the choice to sit it out or dance

I hope you dance...

there are times when

i feel my soul stretching

stirred into wakefulness

by an inner calling

insistent on breaking through

old confinements

and courageously expanding into

more spacious possibilities.

there are times when

like the snake shedding its skin

like the crab molting

like the seed cracking its hull

i too must not cling too long

to an old protective shell

which no longer serves life

my life

lest i be encased in

a prison of my own making

there are times when

uncertain and undefended

i must blindly trust

some deep eternal rhythm

releasing my old self

my old ways of seeing the world

in order to glimpse what's next

there are times when

my next self must wait

naked and vulnerable

in the shadows

and

there are times when

i must expose that hidden self

to the harshest

elements of life

pushing up and through

that which would confine me

so that i can

like the chrysalis

spread my wings and fly

-— 99 Poetic Journeys by Minx Boren -

VALERIE RAMSEY
Biography

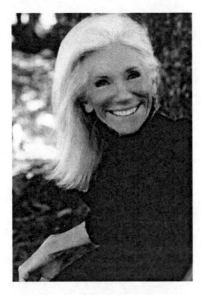

Valerie Ramsey authored her first book, *Gracefully—Looking & Being Your Best at Any Age,* and now has given us her newest updated book—**Creating What's Next—Gracefully.** For many years she was a stay-at-home wife and mother of six. Then, in her 50's, she and her husband moved cross-country to Pebble Beach, CA., where she began a 15-year corporate career as public relations director with the famed Pebble Beach Resorts. At 63, while overseeing a television show on the Pebble Beach Golf Links, she was discovered by a Hollywood producer and subsequently recruited by a major San Francisco modeling agency.

Now in her 70's, Valerie is a strong believer in the importance of being engaged in life and not being afraid to try new things. She is represented by Wilhelmina Models in Miami and New York as well as agencies in Toronto and Paris. Valerie is with Premier Speakers Bureau and travels all over the country to share what she has learned about how to discover What's Next in her own life, and how you can too.

Valerie has been a popular guest on numerous TV shows including several appearances on the TODAY Show, Fox News and Extra.

CPSIA information can be obtained at www.ICGtesting.com
Printed in the USA
LVOW10s1339270514

387402LV00002B/237/P

9 780988 225091